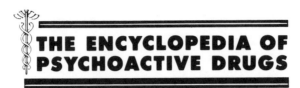

THE ENCYCLOPEDIA OF PSYCHOACTIVE DRUGS

SERIES 1

The Addictive Personality
Alcohol and Alcoholism
Alcohol: *Customs and Rituals*
Alcohol: *Teenage Drinking*
Amphetamines: *Danger in the Fast Lane*
Barbiturates: *Sleeping Potions or Intoxicants?*
Caffeine: *The Most Popular Stimulant*
Cocaine: *A New Epidemic*
Escape from Anxiety and Stress
Flowering Plants: *Magic in Bloom*
Getting Help: *Treatments for Drug Abuse*
Heroin: *The Street Narcotic*
Inhalants: *The Toxic Fumes*

LSD: *Visions or Nightmares?*
Marijuana: *Its Effects on Mind & Body*
Methadone: *Treatment for Addiction*
Mushrooms: *Psychedelic Fungi*
Nicotine: *An Old-Fashioned Addiction*
Over-The-Counter Drugs: *Harmless or Hazardous?*
PCP: *The Dangerous Angel*
Prescription Narcotics: *The Addictive Painkillers*
Quaaludes: *The Quest for Oblivion*
Teenage Depression and Drugs
Treating Mental Illness
Valium: *and Other Tranquilizers*

SERIES 2

Bad Trips
Brain Function
Case Histories
Celebrity Drug Use
Designer Drugs
The Downside of Drugs
Drinking, Driving, and Drugs
Drugs and Civilization
Drugs and Crime
Drugs and Diet
Drugs and Disease
Drugs and Emotion
Drugs and Pain
Drugs and Perception
Drugs and Pregnancy
Drugs and Sexual Behavior

Drugs and Sleep
Drugs and Sports
Drugs and the Arts
Drugs and the Brain
Drugs and the Family
Drugs and the Law
Drugs and Women
Drugs of the Future
Drugs Through the Ages
Drug Use Around the World
Legalization: *A Debate*
Mental Disturbances
Nutrition and the Brain
The Origins and Sources of Drugs
Substance Abuse: *Prevention and Treatment*
Who Uses Drugs?

PCP

EDITOR, WRITER
OF UPDATED MATERIAL

Ann Keene

GENERAL EDITOR
OF UPDATING PROJECT

Professor Paul R. Sanberg, Ph.D.

Department of Psychiatry, Neurosurgery,
Physiology, and Biophysics
University of Cincinnati College of Medicine; and
Director of Neuroscience, Cellular Transplants, Inc.

GENERAL EDITOR

Professor Solomon H. Snyder, M.D.

Distinguished Service Professor of
Neuroscience, Pharmacology, and Psychiatry at
The Johns Hopkins University School of Medicine

ASSOCIATE EDITOR

Professor Barry L. Jacobs, Ph.D.

Program in Neuroscience, Department of Psychology,
Princeton University

SENIOR EDITORIAL CONSULTANT

Jerome H. Jaffe, M.D.

Director of The Addiction Research Center,
National Institute on Drug Abuse

THE ENCYCLOPEDIA OF PSYCHOACTIVE DRUGS

PCP

The Dangerous Angel

MARILYN CARROLL, Ph.D.
University of Minnesota

CHELSEA HOUSE PUBLISHERS
NEW YORK   PHILADELPHIA

Chelsea House Publishers

EDITOR-IN-CHIEF: Remmel Nunn
MANAGING EDITOR: Karyn Gullen Browne
PICTURE EDITOR: Adrian G. Allen
ART DIRECTOR: Maria Epes
MANUFACTURING MANAGER: Gerald Levine
SYSTEMS MANAGER: Lindsey Ottman
PRODUCTION MANAGER: Joseph Romano

THE ENCYCLOPEDIA OF PSYCHOACTIVE DRUGS
EDITOR OF UPDATED MATERIAL: Ann Keene

STAFF FOR PCP: THE DANGEROUS ANGEL
PRODUCTION EDITOR: Marie Claire Cebrián
LAYOUT: Bernard Schleifer
APPENDIXES AND TABLES: Gary Tong
PICTURE RESEARCH: Susan Quist, Toby Greenberg
COVER PHOTO: Frank Lusk

UPDATED 1992
3 5 7 9 8 6 4 2

Library of Congress Cataloging in Publication Data
Carroll, Marilyn.
  PCP, the dangerous angel.
  (Encyclopedia of psychoactive drugs)
  Bibliography: p.
  Includes index.
  Summary: Describes the chemical properties of phencyclidine, or PCP, and its
original use as a presurgery anesthetic. Also discusses the physical and
psychological effects of this hallucinogen, which can cause serious mental illness
and even death.
  1. Phencyclidine abuse—Juvenile literature. 2. Phencyclidine—Toxicology—
Juvenile literature.
  [1. Phencyclidine. 2. Drugs. 3. Drug abuse] I. Title. II. Series.
RC568.P45C37   1985   615'.7883   85-3730'
ISBN 0-87754-753-X
    0-7910-0770-7 (pbk.)

Photos courtesy of Boehringer Ingelheim Animal Health, Inc.; Elaine Mayas;
Museum of the City of New York; National Park Service; Phoenix House; *Press
Telegram*/Bob Amaral, Ann Bailie, Leo Hetzel, & Tom Shaw; Susan Quist; RAP,
Inc.; U.S. Drug Enforcement Agency; UPI/Bettmann Archive; The *Washington
Star*, D.C. Public Library; Wide World Photos, Inc.

CONTENTS

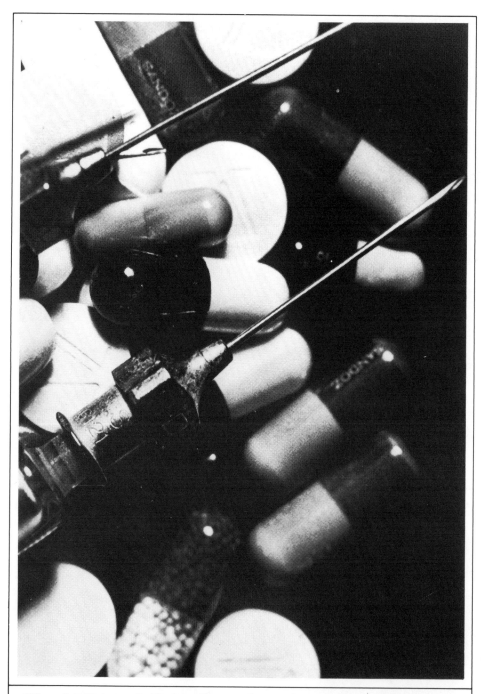

Although PCP is available in tablets and capsules as well as in powder form, it is most commonly sold as a liquid. Liquid PCP is usually applied to a leafy material, such as marijuana, oregano, parsley, or mint, and smoked.

FOREWORD

Since the 1960s, the abuse of psychoactive substances—drugs that alter mood and behavior—has grown alarmingly. Many experts in the fields of medicine, public health, law enforcement, and crime prevention are calling the situation an epidemic. Some legal psychoactive substances—alcohol, caffeine, and nicotine, for example—have been in use since colonial times; illegal ones such as heroin and marijuana have been used to a varying extent by certain segments of the population for decades. But only in the late 20th century has there been widespread reliance on such a variety of mind-altering substances—by youth as well as by adults.

Day after day, newspapers, magazines, and television and radio programs bring us the grim consequences of this dependence. Addiction threatens not only personal health but the stability of our communities and currently costs society an estimated $180 billion annually in the United States alone. Drug-related violent crime and death are increasingly becoming a way of life in many of our cities, towns, and rural areas alike.

Why do people use drugs of any kind? There is one simple answer: to "feel better," physically or mentally. The antibiotics your doctor prescribes for an ear infection destroy the bacteria and make the pain go away. Aspirin can make us more comfortable by reducing fever, banishing a headache, or relieving joint pain from arthritis. Cigarettes put smokers at ease in social situations; a beer or a cocktail helps a worker relax after a hard day on the job. Caffeine, the most widely used drug in America, wakes us up in the morning and overcomes fatigue when we have exams to study for or a long drive to make. Prescription drugs, over-the-counter remedies, tobacco products, alcoholic beverages, caffeine products— all of these are legally available substances that have the capacity to change the way we feel.

But the drugs causing the most concern today are not found in a package of NoDoz or in an aspirin bottle. The drugs that government and private agencies are spending billions of dollars to overcome in the name of crime prevention, law enforcement, rehabilitation, and education have names like crack, angel dust, pot, horse, and speed. Cocaine, PCP, marijuana, heroin, and amphetamines can be very dangerous indeed, to both users and those with whom they live, go to school, and work. But other mood- and mind-altering substances are having a devastating impact, too—especially on youth.

Consider alcohol: The minimum legal drinking age in all 50 states is now 21, but adolescent consumption remains high, even as a decline in other forms of drug use is reported. A recent survey of high school seniors reveals that on any given weekend one in three seniors will be drunk; more than half of all high school seniors report that they have driven while they were drunk. The average age at which a child has his or her first drink is now 12, and more than 1 in 3 eighth-graders report having been drunk at least once.

Or consider nicotine, the psychoactive and addictive ingredient of tobacco: While smoking has declined in the population as a whole, the number of adolescent girls who smoke has been steadily increasing. Because certain health hazards of smoking have been conclusively demonstrated—its relationship to heart disease, lung cancer, and respiratory disease; its link to premature birth and low birth weight of babies whose mothers smoked during pregnancy—the long-term effects of such a trend are a cause for concern.

Studies have shown that almost all drug abuse begins in the preteen and teenage years. It is not difficult to understand why: Adolescence is a time of tremendous change and turmoil, when teenagers face the tasks of discovering their identity, clarifying their sexual roles, asserting their independence as they learn to cope with authority, and searching for goals. The pressures—from friends, parents, teachers, coaches, and one's own self—are great, and the temptation to want to "feel better" by taking drugs is powerful.

Psychoactive drugs are everywhere in our society, and their use and misuse show no sign of waning. The lack of success in the so-called war on drugs, begun in earnest in the 1980s, has shown us that we cannot "drug proof" our homes, schools, workplaces, and communities. What we can do, however, is make available the latest information on these substances and their effects and ask that those reading it consider the information carefully.

The newly updated ENCYCLOPEDIA OF PSYCHOACTIVE DRUGS, specifically written for young people, provides up-to-date information on a variety of substances that are widely abused in today's society. Each volume is devoted to a specific substance or pattern of abuse and is designed to answer the questions that young readers are likely to ask about drugs. An individualized glossary in each volume defines key words and terms, and newly enlarged and updated appendixes include recent statistical data as well as a special section on AIDS and its relation to drug abuse. The editors of the ENCYCLOPEDIA OF PSYCHOACTIVE DRUGS hope this series will help today's adolescents make intelligent choices as they prepare for maturity in the 21st century.

Ann Keene, Editor

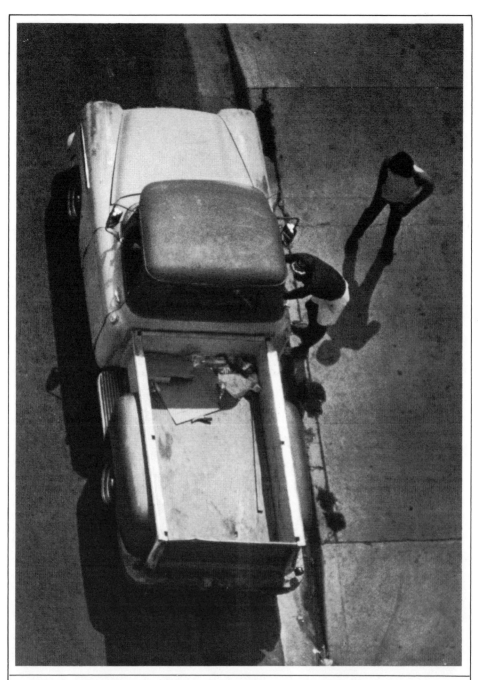

A drug deal transpires not far from the Capitol in Washington, D.C. In 1988, 42% of all PCP-related hospital emergency room admissions nationwide occurred in Washington, which has the dubious distinction of being the "PCP capital" of the United States.

INTRODUCTION

USES AND ABUSES

JACK H. MENDELSON, M.D.
NANCY K. MELLO, Ph.D.
Alcohol and Drug Abuse Research Center
Harvard Medical School—McLean Hospital

*H*uman beings are endowed with the gift of wizardry, a talent for discovery and invention. The discovery and invention of substances that change the way we feel and behave are among our special accomplishments, and like so many other products of our wizardry, these substances have the capacity to harm as well as to help.

Consider alcohol—available to all and recognized as both harmful and pleasure inducing since biblical times. The use of alcoholic beverages dates back to our earliest ancestors. Alcohol use and misuse became associated with the worship of gods and demons. One of the most powerful Greek gods was Dionysus, lord of fruitfulness and god of wine. The Romans adopted Dionysus but changed his name to Bacchus. Festivals and holidays associated with Bacchus celebrated the harvest and the origins of life. Time has blurred the images of the Bacchanalian festival, but the theme of drunkenness as a major part of celebration has survived the pagan gods and remains a familiar part of modern society. The term *Bacchanalian festival* conveys a more appealing image than "drunken orgy" or "pot party," but whatever the label, some of the celebrants will inevitably start up the "high" escalator to the next plateau. Once there, the de-escalation is often difficult.

According to reliable estimates, 1 out of every 10 Americans develops a serious alcohol-related problem sometime in his or her lifetime. In addition, automobile accidents caused by drunken drivers claim the lives of more than 20,000 people each year, and injure 25 times that number. Many of the victims are gifted young people just starting out in adult life. Hospital emergency rooms abound with patients seeking help for alcohol-related injuries.

Who is to blame? Can we blame the many manufacturers who produce such an amazing variety of alcoholic beverages? Should we blame the educators who fail to explain the perils of intoxication or so exaggerate the dangers of drinking that no one could possibly believe them? Are friends to blame— those peers who urge others to "drink more and faster," or the macho types who stress the importance of being able to "hold your liquor?" Casting blame, however, is hardly constructive, and pointing the finger is a fruitless way to deal with problems. Alcoholism and drug abuse have few culprits but many victims. Accountability begins with each of us, every time we choose to use or to misuse an intoxicating substance.

It is ironic that some of our earliest medicines, derived from natural plant products, are used today to poison and to intoxicate. Relief from pain and suffering is one of society's many continuing goals. More than 3,000 years ago, the Therapeutic Papyrus of Thebes, one of our earliest written records, gave instructions for the use of opium in the treatment of pain. Opium, in the form of its major derivative, morphine, remains one of the most powerful drugs we have for pain relief. But opium, morphine, and similar compounds, such as heroin, have also been used by many to induce changes in mood and feeling. Another example of a natural substance that has been misused is the coca leaf, which for centuries was used by the Indians of Peru to reduce fatigue and hunger. Its modern derivative, cocaine, has important medical use as a local anesthetic. Unfortunately, its increasing abuse in recent years has reached epidemic proportions.

The purpose of this series is to provide information about the nature and behavioral effects of alcohol and drugs and the probable consequences of their use. The authors believe that up-to-date, objective information about alcohol and drugs will help readers make better decisions about the wisdom of their use. The information presented here (and in other books in this series) is based on many clinical and laboratory studies and observations by people from diverse walks of life.

Over the centuries, novelists, poets, and dramatists have provided us with many insights into the effects of alcohol and drug use. Physicians, lawyers, biologists, psychologists, and social scientists have contributed to a better understanding of the causes and consequences of using these substances. The authors in this series have attempted to gather and condense all the latest information about drug use. They have also described the sometimes wide gaps in our knowledge and have suggested some new ways to answer many difficult questions.

How, for example, do alcohol and drug problems get started? And what is the best way to treat them when they do? Not too many years ago, alcoholics and drug abusers were regarded as evil, immoral, or both. Many now believe that these persons suffer from very complicated diseases involving deep psychological and social problems. To understand how the disease begins and progresses, it is necessary to understand the nature of the substance, the behavior of the afflicted person, and the characteristics of the society or culture in which that person lives.

The diagram below shows the interaction of these three factors. The arrows indicate that the substance not only affects the user personally but the society as well. Society influences attitudes toward the substance, which in turn affect its availability. The substance's impact upon the society may support or discourage the use and abuse of that substance.

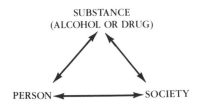

SUBSTANCE
(ALCOHOL OR DRUG)

PERSON ◄────────► SOCIETY

Although many of the social environments we live in are very similar, some of the most subtle differences can strongly influence our thinking and behavior. Where we live, go to school and work, whom we discuss things with—all influence our opinions about drug use. Yet we also share certain commonly accepted beliefs that outweigh any differences in our attitudes. The authors in this series have tried to identify and discuss the central, most crucial issues concerning drug use.

Regrettably, human wizardry in developing new substances in medical therapeutics has not always been paralleled by intelligent usage. Although we do know a great deal about the effects of alcohol and drugs, we have yet to learn how to impart that knowledge, especially to young adults.

Does it matter? What harm does it do to smoke a little pot or have a few beers? What is it like to be intoxicated? How long does it last? Will it make me feel really fine? Will it make me sick? What are the risks? These are but a few of the questions answered in this series, which we hope will enable the reader to make wise decisions concerning the crucial issue of drugs.

Information sensibly acted upon can go a long way toward helping everyone develop his or her best self. As one keen and sensitive observer, Dr. Lewis Thomas, has said,

> *There is nothing at all absurd about the human condition. We matter. It seems to me a good guess, hazarded by a good many people who have thought about it, that we may be engaged in the formation of something like a mind for the life of this planet. If this is so, we are still at the most primitive stage, still fumbling with language and thinking, but infinitely capacitated for the future. Looked at this way, it is remarkable that we've come as far as we have in so short a period, really no time at all as geologists measure time. We are the newest, the youngest, and the brightest thing around.*

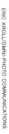

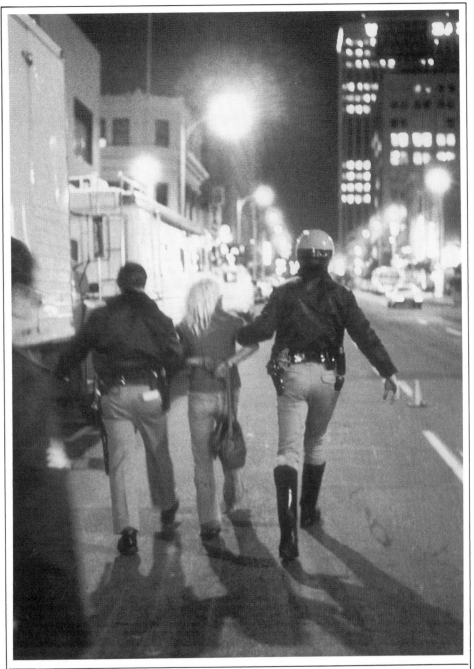

A girl is arrested in San Diego for drug possession. Southern California has long been a center for PCP production. Liquid supplies of the drug not consumed locally are shipped to other areas where PCP is in demand, including New Orleans, Chicago, and Oklahoma City.

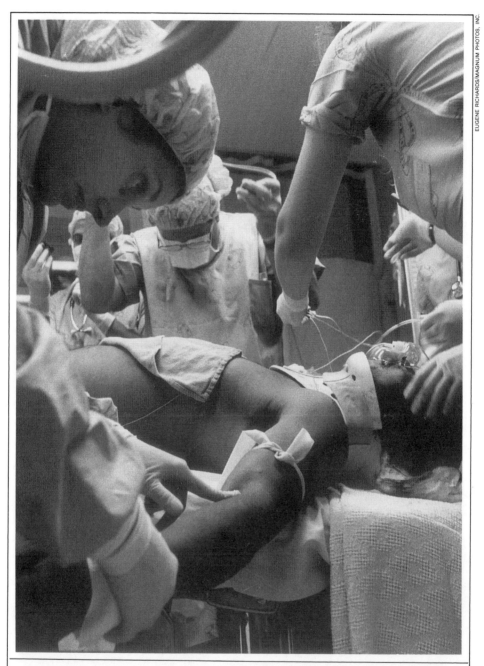

Doctors administer anesthesia to a surgical patient. Phencyclidine—PCP— was originally developed in the late 1950s as a human anesthetic, but several years of testing revealed that patients became agitated, delusional, and irrational after receiving the drug. Legal human use was discontinued in 1965.

CHAPTER 1

WHAT IS PCP?

PCP goes by many names—angel dust, crystal, peace pill, and loveboat, to name a few. In fact, police files show that the more unusual the street name of a drug, the more likely it will prove to be phencyclidine, the scientific name for one of the newer recreational drugs.

The great variety of names given to PCP reflects the great diversity of its effects. While it can sometimes produce pleasurable feelings, it can also create strange and unpleasant ones. News reports of the bizarre and often violent behavior that accompanied the use of PCP gave it a bad reputation even within the drug culture. It first appeared as a street drug in 1967 but quickly lost favor and was replaced by other drugs. In the mid-1970s, it regained its popularity as a street drug among young adults, but horror stories about the drug's effects again led to a decline in its use, at least among the middle-class population. In the 1990s, however, PCP continues to be a problem in major U.S. cities.

On the street PCP is often substituted for other drugs, so users frequently do not know they are taking it. Drugs sold as methamphetamine (speed), mescaline, psilocybin (psychedelic mushrooms), LSD, and THC (tetra-hydrocannabinol, the psychoactive ingredient in marijuana) frequently prove to be PCP. Actual THC is exceedingly unstable and is thus very rare. In nearly every case in which a sample of supposed

THC was confiscated, laboratory results showed that it was really PCP. This confusion of PCP with other drugs and its unknowing use often results in unforeseen and frightening consequences.

In one case, a 38-year-old man who had smoked marijuana regularly bought something that was said to be "superweed." Once he started using it he became paranoid, delusional, and hostile. He decided the new drug was responsible and stopped taking it. When his symptoms failed to subside, he returned to the drug and actually increased the dose, hoping to relieve his symptoms. As it turned out, this only aggravated the symptoms. He became extremely aggressive, decapitated his dog, and attacked a stranger with a razor. When his girlfriend brought him to the hospital, the doctors who examined him discovered that his marijuana was laced with PCP. After a brief hospitalization, during which he received antipsychotic medication, he refused further treatment. Following his discharge, he continued with supportive counseling.

Street Names for PCP: A Partial List

Since the appearance of phencyclidine (PCP) as a street drug in the late 1960s, it has been sold under at least 100 different names. The following is a list of some of the more popular—and lasting—ones:

angel dust	mist
animal tranquilizer	Mr. Lovely
black death	peace pill
crystal	the pits
DOA	rocket fuel
dust	Shermans
elephant tranquilizer	street drug
embalming fluid	supergrass
hog	superweed
horse tranquilizer	tea
jet fuel	THC
killer weed	tranq
krystal joint (KJ)	wacky weed
loveboat ('boat)	whack
lovely	

Although his psychotic symptoms faded after two weeks, he continued to complain of impaired thinking, prolonged depression, and difficulty in believing that the delusions that he perceived during his PCP intoxication were imaginary. After several months of supportive counseling, these symptoms apparently faded.

This widespread masking of PCP makes it difficult to study the drug because users' reports are often inaccurate sources of information. Fortunately for researchers, the unique effects of PCP usually make it identifiable even in the absence of reliable user information.

Unlike many other abused drugs, such as cocaine, heroin, or marijuana, PCP is not derived from or related to any natural base, but is completely synthetic. Because PCP is easily manufactured, its distribution and use present unusual economic and legal complications.

Early Medical Use of PCP

Phencyclidine was commercially developed in the late 1950s by Parke, Davis & Company as an intravenous anesthetic named Serynl (derived from the word serenity). Early tests on animals indicated that the drug might be very useful in surgery both as an anesthetic (to cause physical insensibility) and as an analgesic (a pain killer).

In 1964, when the federal government allowed the manufacturers to test the drug on humans, PCP promised to be the ideal anesthetic. It did not affect breathing, it relieved pain, and it mildly stimulated the heart. Thus, it appeared to satisfy important surgical needs.

Based on experiments using monkeys as subjects, PCP was found to have a high therapeutic ratio. This important indicator is calculated by dividing the amount needed to cause death by the minimum needed to produce the desired effect. Most commonly used general anesthetics have a therapeutic ratio close to 2. That of PCP was found to be 26.

While with other drugs the difference between fatal overdose and the amount needed to sedate safely is small, and the chance of administering too much is thus great, PCP seemed to be a very safe drug. The amount that would cause a lethal overdose was 26 times the amount needed to sedate the patient. Another advantage of PCP from the surgeon's point of view was that, unlike other anesthetics, it did not suppress activity of the entire nervous system. Rather, it only blocked the sensation of pain. Throughout the early 1960s the drug was tested on hospital patients to calm them before surgery, to eliminate pain and sensation during surgery, to relieve pain after surgery, and to control unbearable pain such as that suffered by severe burn victims.

The Discovery of PCP's Side Effects

Unfortunately, medical hopes for PCP began to diminish when increasing numbers of hospital patients reported post-surgical symptoms of confusion, terror, and unpleasant hallucinations. The hallucinations did not resemble the visual distortions produced by LSD, but involved perceptual distortions of the body image, feelings of separation of the body from the environment, and occasional sensations of weightlessness.

Doctors and researchers began to doubt the usefulness of PCP as an anesthetic. Researchers began to focus on the drug's psychoactive properties, creating ways to measure its effects on behavior. To do this PCP was tested on several thousand volunteers in prisons, colleges, and hospitals. Because of its negative effects, however, tests were stopped in 1965. Until 1979 phencyclidine continued to be manufactured by Bio-Ceutic Laboratories, Inc., for use as an anesthetic for animals, with its name changed to Sernylan. At the present time it is carefully regulated by the government. It can be used only for animal research and cannot be administered to humans for any purpose. Today PCP is only manufactured by the federal government for distribution to licensed researchers. All other production is strictly illegal.

When phencyclidine first appeared on the streets of San Francisco in the late 1960s, it was known as the "peace pill" (PeaCe Pill). Shortly afterward, its appearance was reported in New York's Greenwich Village. When PCP was taken as a pill, users had difficulty controlling the doses necessary to obtain only pleasant effects. Many users suffered frightening symptoms. PCP's low cost, however, made it an attractive substitute for other consciousness-altering drugs such as THC, cocaine, mescaline, and psychedelic mushrooms.

Although PCP produces some of the positive effects of these other drugs, its negative effects greatly contributed to its bad reputation. PCP tablets disappeared from the streets by the late 1960s after the publication of well-documented news stories which described the bizarre behavior that often accompanied the drug's use.

Within a few years PCP resurfaced in a form which found greater favor inside the drug culture. In 1972 it became available as a liquid or powder, which could easily be added to parsley, mint, oregano, tea, tobacco, or marijuana and smoked.

The PCP users of the 1970s were also different from those who rejected the drug the previous decade. Many of the new users turned to PCP to boost the effects of marijuana, or because of their interest in mood-altering sedatives or stimulants. In this last respect, they were unlike the PCP users of the 1960s, who were mainly interested in hallucinogenic experiences.

The fact that PCP could now be smoked contributed to its rise in popularity in two ways: it was now easier to control the dosage and thus avoid overdose, and the onset of the effects of the drug was more rapid than when it was taken in pill form.

In the 1970s PCP clearly gained its own identity, though drug dealers continued to represent it as a variety of other substances. In the reports of the Drug Abuse Warning Network (DAWN) from 1972 to 1975, PCP use increased rapidly, pushing it from twenty-third to fifth place on the statistical scale of abused drugs. The popularity of PCP declined somewhat toward the end of the decade, and by 1981 it had fallen to tenth place. Another wave of increase occurred during the 1980s, and by 1988 PCP again ranked fifth in DAWN's list of drugs mentioned most frequently in reports from hospital emergency rooms across the country. (See Appendices II and III for a summary of 1988 DAWN data. For more information on DAWN, see also Chapter 6, "Who Uses PCP?"

The Physical Appearance of PCP

In its pure form PCP is a white crystalline powder that readily dissolves in water or alcohol. It has a distinctive bitter taste. Most PCP contains contaminants resulting from its haphazard manufacture, causing the color to range from tan to brown and the consistency to range from a powder to a gummy mass. Because PCP mixes easily with dyes, it has turned up on the illicit drug market in a variety of tablets, capsules, and colored powders. During the 1980s PCP became increasingly available on the street as a liquid, which was applied to marijuana, parsley, or other plant leaves and smoked; although injection is possible, PCP is rarely used today in this way. Smoking toothpick-sized "joints" of PCP-sprayed marijuana, known on the street as "loveboat," is now the most common form of PCP use.

Classifying PCP

The term "dissociative anesthesia" refers to a state in which a person is aware of physical sensations (touch, pressure, or pain) but they are not interpreted as such by the brain. This is why patients who were anesthetized with PCP during hospital studies reported feelings of unreality. They were wakeful, but scarcely moved from rigidly held positions. They were aware of their environment but did not feel they were part of it.

Other commonly used anesthetics block all sensations from reaching the brain. Conventional barbiturate anesthetics put the patient into a sleepy, relaxed, hypnotic state. The initial appeal of PCP as an anesthetic was that, unlike other anesthetics, at moderate doses it did not suppress breathing and heart rate. Until the adverse side effects were known, researchers felt they had uncovered a valuable new surgical aid.

Phencyclidine is classified by the Drug Enforcement Administration (DEA) as a hallucinogen. But only rarely, and only when taken in large amounts, does it produce the vivid, colorful hallucinations characteristic of drugs such as LSD or mescaline. Rather, the distortions of body image and feelings of separation from the environment that PCP produces are characteristic of a relatively new class of drugs termed *dissociative anesthetics*. PCP is the most typical of this class of drugs, labeled arylcyclohexylamines, which includes cyclohexamine and ketamine, drugs with a similar chemical structure.

The PCP Analogs

There are at least 30 PCP analogs and many of these have appeared in confiscated street samples. (An analog is a drug that is similar to another drug in both chemical structure and function.) Since the only street source of PCP is illegal manufacture (often by amateur chemists and in labs with no quality control), there is always a good chance that analogs rather than pure PCP will be produced and sold. The manufacture of PCP involves the use of potentially dangerous or volatile chemicals such as ether, benzene, potassium cyanide, and hydrochloric acid. Because improper synthesis can create PCP analogs, information about the analogs is important, for some have poisonous by-products which might be lethal to the unsuspecting PCP user. For example, the PCP analog known as PCC can produce cyanide in the blood of the user, causing bloody vomiting, diarrhea, and abdominal cramps. Such symptoms would clearly indicate that the drug user had ingested the more dangerous analog PCC.

Ketamine, the only PCP analog that can be produced legally, is similar to PCP in most respects, but only about one-tenth to one-twentieth as potent, depending upon the effect that is being measured. It has more depressant properties than PCP, and is shorter acting. It is used for surgical anesthesia in high-risk patients, such as the very young or old, and is also the preferred drug for burn victims.

Several PCP analogs have appeared in street samples. Ketamine has been found in capsules and in stolen vials of the injectable solution used for human and veterinary anesthesia. In 1969 another analog, PCE, similar to PCP in potency and duration of action, appeared on the streets of Los Angeles. Another analog, TCP, was first seen in 1972, and by 1975 its use had spread to many areas of the West Coast and to 22 states. TCP is more potent and shorter acting than PCP. Since the government placed restrictions on piperidine, an essential ingredient in the production of PCP analogs, the analog PHP has been produced by street chemists. Other analogs such as NPPCA and PCPY have also surfaced. The results of studies with animals suggest that all these analogs are likely to be as widely abused as PCP itself.

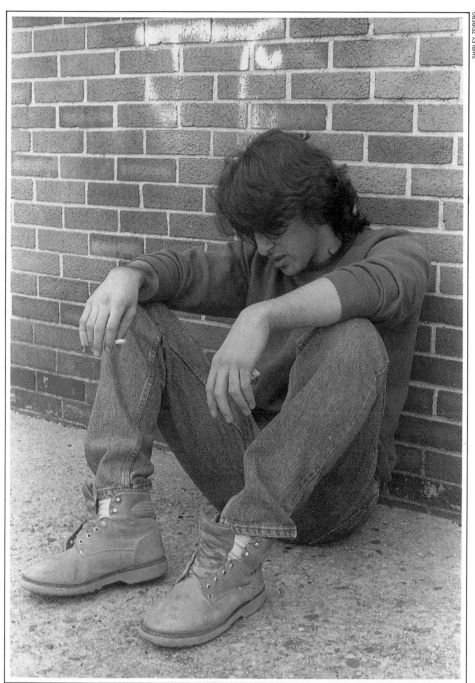

SHIRLEY ZEIBERG

Although physical and emotional reactions related to the use of PCP vary depending on the dosage and the personality of the user, it is generally characteristic of the PCP user to experience a degree of amnesia, or loss of memory.

CHAPTER 2

THE EFFECTS OF PCP

*T*he feelings or moods brought on by the use of drugs produce what is known as the subjective experience. Perceptual and emotional reactions to PCP vary widely depending upon the user's personality, the amount of the drug taken, whether or not there is a family history of mental disturbance, and the user's expectations, usually based upon past drug experiences. And because of the great range of possible reactions to PCP, users can experience vastly different results on different occasions. One characteristic of PCP is to produce a certain degree of amnesia (loss of memory). Thus far there have been no studies to determine if this amnesia is different for those experiencing positive effects from those experiencing negative effects. Nor is it known if amnesia is related to the amount of PCP taken.

One study, which only varied the dosage of PCP, described the feelings of the users. A low dose (5 milligrams or less) typically produces effects which begin within a few minutes, peak in 30 minutes, and last for four to six hours. The effects of PCP on mood are usually completely gone within 24 hours.

Higher doses (10 milligrams or more) intensify all the low dose effects and produce additional ones. The study is summarized in Table 1.

Table 1

PCP's Effects on Mood, Perception, and Thinking

LOW DOSE
(0–5 mg)
    Mild to intense "high"
    Feelings of unreality
    Feelings of separation from environment
    Distortions in seeing and hearing
    Difficulties in concentrating and thinking
HIGH DOSE
(10 + mg)
    The low-dose effects intensified plus:
    Disorientation
    Confusion
    Restlessness and panic
    Obsession with trivial matters
    Fear of being near death

An unusual effect of PCP is that users may go through the whole spectrum of feelings as the body absorbs greater and greater amounts of the drug. Then, as the body throws off the drug, they may experience them again on the way down from the "high." While the pleasant effects of the "high" may be amplified with higher doses, the number and degree of unpleasant effects are also increased. In fact, in a study of 319 users all reported some negative effects with every use, but experienced positive effects only 60% of the time.

Other studies with smaller numbers of users have confirmed the general finding that fewer than half of the people questioned in the sample report that their typical PCP experience was pleasant. In some studies 50% to 80% of those questioned, however, stated that their first experience with the drug was very positive. Those who initially have a positive experience with PCP appear more likely to develop a pattern of regular use than those whose initial experience was negative.

In a study of 25 PCP users (20 males and 5 females), 80% reported a pleasant high and a sense of numbness after their first experience with PCP. These individuals continued taking the drug and eventually increased their dosage, hoping to re-create their initial positive experience. Though all of the subjects interviewed used PCP, only 56% considered it their favorite drug.

Despite having heard that PCP was a dangerous drug, 24 of the 25 subjects continued to use it. Some had used it for as long as 9 years, though the average was 4.2 years. The average frequency of use was 2.5 times per day, 5.8 days per week. Asked why they continued to take PCP when it often caused negative experiences, the users said they were "unable to stop," and that they were "seeking an occasional positive experience."

The same study also reported that 68% of those who frequently used PCP had been introduced to it by a friend. Even more disturbing is the fact that, although 88% of the group had friends who had suffered severe reactions to PCP, involving injuries, near fatalities, and long periods of psychiatric hospitalization, the knowledge did not deter them from using PCP.

How PCP Changes Behavior

Relatively few experiments have employed objective measures to determine the effects of PCP on human behavior. In such studies, small groups of volunteers were administered oral doses of PCP (5 to 7.5 milligrams) and then subjected

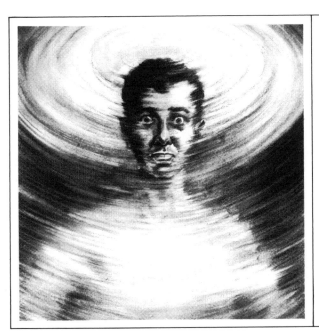

This self-portrait by a schizophrenic patient captures the sense of anxiety and confusion frequently described by those who use PCP. PCP is virtually unique among popular drugs of abuse in its power to produce psychoses often indistinguishable from schizophrenia.

Table 2

PCP's Effects on Behavior	
LOW DOSE (0-5 mg)	HIGH DOSE (10 + mg)

Speech disturbances or no speech
Gross and fine muscular incoordination
Blank stare
Difficulty walking
Blurred vision, dizziness, and drowsiness
Racing thoughts or thinking faster than
    one can talk
Rapid mood changes, anxiety, agitation,
    paranoid thinking, panic, terror, and
    thought disorganization
	Erratic, bizarre, or violent behavior
	Compulsive and repetitive movements
	Incoherent speech
	Severe psychological disorganization
	Paranoia, agitation, and restlessness
	Acute toxic psychosis

to a battery of tests to measure physical and mental performance. The results of these tests revealed that PCP causes alterations in sight, hearing, touch, orientation, memory, attention, and motor function. Most subjects noted that changes in sensation and perception preceded the impairment of their performance in a given task. Other information about the behavioral effects of PCP has been culled from questions asked of PCP users, and from observations of users by the personnel of drug treatment facilities. Table 2 describes the visible behavioral changes resulting from various doses.

Subjective changes take place at the same time as observable changes in mood, feelings, or perceptions; however, the observable changes may lag slightly behind. These observable effects peak at 30 minutes and last from four to six hours.

Ways That PCP Affects the Body

In a hospital no treatment can begin until the staff has determined what is wrong. If a patient does not know or cannot remember what drug he may have taken, doctors must learn whatever they can from his appearance and from the results of certain routine tests.

Patients admitted to hospitals for treatment of PCP will often show some of the effects listed in the low dose column of Table 3. Because rapid vertical eye movement is not commonly associated with other psychoactive drugs, pres-

Table 3

PCP's Effects on the Body	
LOW DOSE (5–10 mg by an occasional user, 5–15 mg by a regular user)	HIGH DOSE (10–20 mg or more)
Muscle rigidity Small, rapid eye movements vertically or horizontally (nystagmus) Excessive water intake and urinary output Decreased sensitivity to pain	Eyes may remain open although rapid horizontal and vertical oscillation is still present Elevated blood pressure alternating with abnormally low blood pressure Elevated body temperature Decreased urinary output Slow, shallow, and/or irregular breathing Irregular heartbeat Repeated vomiting Convulsions and coma Death

ence of this symptom could help a medical attendant determine that the patient had taken PCP. However, vertical eye movement may also be a sign of brain damage, so the possibility of accident or trauma cannot be ruled out. Except when massive doses have been taken, PCP does not produce many effects similar to those of other psychoactive drugs. For example, contrary to other drugs, PCP often does not cause abnormalities in heart rate, respiration, and blood pressure. There is also no enlargement or dilation of the pupil as would be noted with patients who had taken cocaine, amphetamine, or LSD.

The results of higher doses of PCP (10 to 20 milligrams or more) are also shown in Table 3. Of the possible effects of large doses, death or coma is the most serious. The coma may last from hours to days. During recovery from a coma, which may take at least several days, some of the physiological effects described for lower doses appear.

A case study may help clarify the different ways in which people respond to similar amounts of PCP. At a rock concert in the San Francisco Bay area, six adolescents took an unknown quantity of PCP in tablet form. They had previously smoked PCP in the form of "joints," but this was the first time they had taken tablets. All six became highly intoxicated. Five recovered quickly, but one, a 17-year-old white male high school senior, went into a coma. Friends took him to the local hospital emergency room. His breathing was shallow and all his muscles were extremely rigid. Hospital staff kept him on a respirator for three days. Subsequently, he remained in the hospital in a confused state for about a week. During this time he suffered memory loss and depression. With supportive management, however, he eventually recovered.

Drugs Used in Combination with PCP

Compared with other drug users, PCP users are more likely to abuse other substances, either alternating or combining other drugs with PCP. Before 1974 PCP was frequently mixed with LSD. During the late seventies and early eighties, alcohol was PCP's most frequent accompaniment, when the drug was commonly taken in pill or powdered form. Today PCP is most often used in conjunction with marijuana. This combination, as noted earlier, is known as "loveboat" and is created when PCP is sprayed on marijuana leaves; they are then smoked as "joints."

While the observed effects of "loveboat" are reported as similar to those of other forms of PCP use—ranging from disorientation to death—and are thought to increase in severity as the amount of PCP is increased, scientific studies of this and other PCP combinations in humans are difficult to perform. PCP can cause amnesia, and users are often unable to remember what other drugs they may have taken. A further difficulty is that PCP is sometimes sold as another substance such as THC or mescaline, and even when it is sold as PCP, the dose is seldom pure but is mixed with unknown adulterants or other drugs. Dealers in Washington, D.C., for example, have reportedly combined PCP with formaldehyde and roach spray to give it a more "chemical" odor.

Parallels with Animal Reactions

The effects of PCP on people have been determined primarily from users' reports and from scientific observation. As it is now illegal to test PCP on humans, data must be collected from animals.

There have been several well-designed and controlled studies, using monkeys as subjects, that provide more exact profiles of the effects of PCP. Since studies using monkey and human subjects consistently show that the two groups respond to drugs similarly, it can be assumed that the results of PCP research utilizing monkeys may also apply to humans. In differing degrees research with other animals can also prove informative.

In rats, mice, and guinea pigs low doses of PCP result in increased motor activity, while higher doses produce typically drug-associated behavior such as running in circles around the cage, and continuous swaying of the head. Very high doses produce a marked loss of coordination (ataxia). In monkeys, very low doses may produce a slight increase in the rate of activity, while low to moderate doses often result

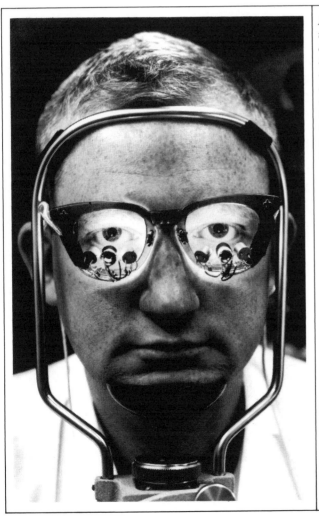

In treating possible victims of PCP use, doctors often use tests that measure patients' eye movements. This device uses photoelectric cells to translate such movements into electric signals which, with the aid of a computer, can then be analyzed.

in mild sedation and a slight loss of coordination. High doses may produce severe motor problems, anesthesia, and/or convulsions.

As researchers work their way up the hierarchy of animal subjects, from rats, mice, and guinea pigs, to cats and dogs, to monkeys, and finally to humans, smaller amounts (per unit of body weight) of PCP are needed to produce anesthesia. Obviously, then, PCP has a greater effect on animals with more highly developed brains.

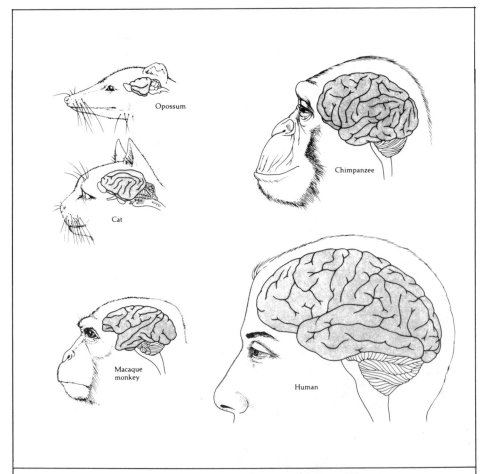

Opossum

Chimpanzee

Cat

Macaque monkey

Human

Research has demonstrated that as one climbs the evolutionary ladder, and the brain becomes more complex and highly developed, smaller doses of PCP per unit of body weight are needed to produce anesthesia.

Studies have also revealed that PCP severely reduces the performance of experimental animals in tests concerned with learning, memory, and motor coordination. The drug may also interfere with an animal's ability to obtain such necessities as food or water, or to avoid punishment (electric shock, for example).

Studies with squirrel monkeys, rats, and mice have generally shown that in small doses PCP does not cause aggressive behavior. In larger doses it decreases aggression, just as it reduces other levels of behavior. More experiments will be necessary to discover the combination of factors that have produced visibly aggressive behavior in humans who have taken PCP.

Animals will voluntarily take most drugs that humans abuse, with the exception of LSD and THC. Rhesus monkeys will accept PCP either orally or intravenously. Some monkeys have taken PCP daily for several years with no apparent damage to any of the organ systems. When the monkeys can obtain PCP during only part of the day (three hours), no severe effects have been noted; about 45 minutes after a high oral dose the monkeys lose coordination, salivate excessively, and move their eyes horizontally and vertically very rapidly. They usually recover completely within four to six hours. However, monkeys performed poorly when they were required to push a lever to receive unlimited intravenous injections of PCP. They became incapable of eating and, at times, injured themselves. Some even overdosed and died.

Laboratory tests which allow animals to choose whether or not to take a drug have proved useful in isolating the factors that influence degree of interest in a drug. For example, as the available amount of PCP is increased, animals take more. However, if they have to work harder for each dose of PCP, the amount taken tends to decrease. When drugs similar to PCP are substituted, they are as readily consumed. Other drugs such as amphetamine or methohexital (a sedative) may be substituted for PCP, and are found to yield similar results.

A significant finding is that animals are much more likely to begin taking drugs when they are deprived of food or another positive aspect of their environment. Conversely, the introduction of another rewarding substance (such as a sweet drink) or an unlimited supply of food greatly reduces the amount of PCP monkeys take. The results of the animal studies imply that people may be more likely to take PCP in an environment that is lacking in other rewards, although this has not been statistically confirmed.

Studies have also been conducted to determine whether animals are capable of distinguishing between the effects of PCP and other drugs. If PCP truly represents a completely separate class of drugs, one would expect animals to be capable of discriminating between it and other drugs.

In one discrimination test a monkey was trained to press one lever after the experimenter injected it with PCP, and another lever when it was injected with a saline solution (which produces no effect). Selection of the appropriate lever was rewarded with food, water, or postponement of electric shock. When the monkey had mastered this, other test drugs were then substituted for PCP. If the monkey consistently selected the lever it had been taught to associate with PCP, this would suggest that the animal considered the other drug similar to PCP. If the animal showed no

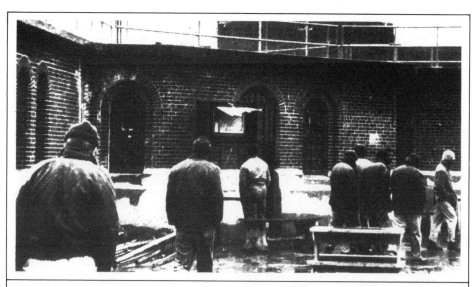

Inmates at Attica prison in upstate New York. Police records show that PCP use can lead to conviction for violent acts—an immense price to pay for a "high" that is unpredictable and often unpleasant.

consistent lever preference, randomly selecting levers, or always chose the saline lever, it could be assumed that the effects of the test drugs were different from PCP. By varying the dose of the test drugs and the PCP, it was also possible to determine the potency of the test drugs in comparison with that of PCP.

From such drug-discrimination tests it was shown that three chemical classes of drugs produce effects similar to those of PCP. These are arylcyclohexylamines (cyclohexamine, ketamine, PCE, PCM, PHP, TCP, and other PCP analogs); opium derivatives; and the dioxolans (dexoxydrol and etoxydrol). In similar tests amphetamine, pentobarbital, THC, and LSD were shown to produce effects unlike those of PCP.

Another finding from animal studies relates to human drug dependence and the powerful effects of the stimuli associated with self-administered drugs. Studies with PCP and monkeys have shown that the taste of the drug, the click of the drinking dispenser, the lights signaling PCP availability, and the tactile (touch) sensation of liquid in the mouth all become associated with the "rewarding" effects of

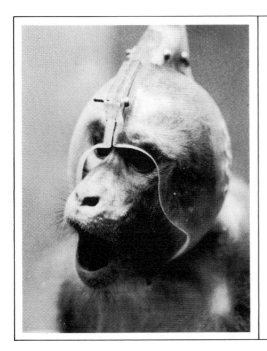

Resembling a junior astronaut, this rhesus monkey awaits his laboratory dose of PCP. PCP's effects vary by species. Monkeys given large doses are at first calm, and then become anesthetized enough to allow painless surgery. Dogs, however, yelp and go into convulsions. At low doses monkeys are serene, while mice become agitated and never become anesthetized. Research has found that a human's response to this drug is similar to a monkey's.

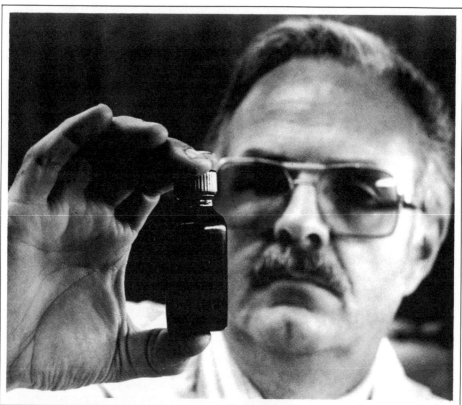

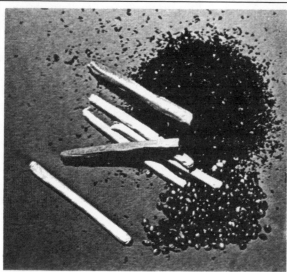

A police officer displays a bottle of liquid PCP. Marijuana is often treated with PCP and rolled into toothpick-sized "joints" (left) for smoking. This marijuana-PCP combination, known as "loveboat," can be powerful and, literally, deadly: fatalities have been reported from its use.

PCP. Even when PCP is no longer available, these stimuli can trigger a considerable amount of drug-seeking behavior. Presentation of these same stimuli also produces long sequences of behavior leading the animal to a single chance to receive the drug. This directed behavior is similar to the complex sequence of behaviors people exhibit while purchasing, taking, and experiencing a drug.

A similar situation occurs when people who have entered a drug-treatment facility stop taking drugs and return to their old environment. The people, places, and paraphernalia (equipment) previously associated with drug-taking often lead the former user to resume the drug-taking habit.

As with other studies of the effects of PCP, its effects in combination with other drugs have been most clearly established in laboratory studies using animals. PCP generally increases the effects of sedatives such as the barbiturates and alcohol. In mice the number of deaths from pentobarbital increased when PCP was added.

In rats PCP increases those movements typically caused by amphetamine. And in both rats and mice PCP adds to the disruptive effects of THC on various learning and motor tasks. While a combination of PCP and THC decreased spontaneous motor activity in mice, THC alone produced no effect, and PCP alone increased activity. In monkeys pentobarbital at low doses increased the disruptive effects of PCP on food-rewarded behavior. Both pentobarbital and amphetamine increased the amount of PCP that monkeys took, while neither drug increased the intake of a sugar solution. At higher doses the rewarded behavior was suppressed.

Other animal studies suggest that a marijuana/PCP combination has the potential for producing effects different from those produced by PCP alone.

Laboratory studies suggest that the effects of PCP are increased by most other drugs that people abuse. Thus far there have not been scientific studies of the behavioral effects of combining PCP and other commonly used drugs, such as alcohol and nicotine. It is important that research focus on these variables so we can better understand, predict, and treat the effects.

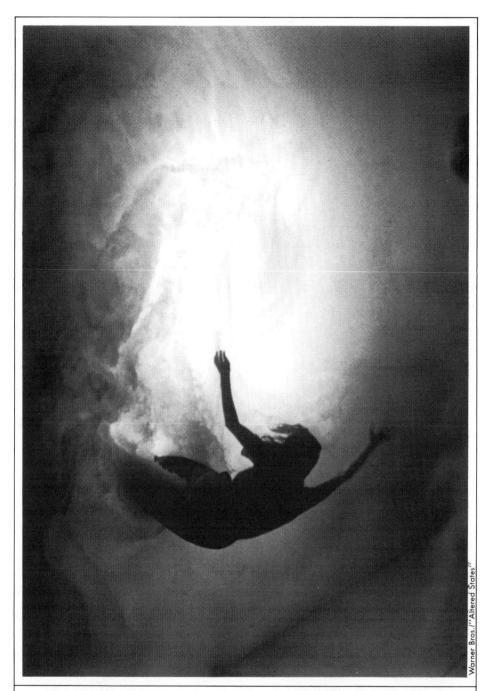

Warner Bros./"Altered States"

At first the sensation of floating produced by PCP may be pleasurable. However, the regular user may suddenly become paranoid and delusional, and suffer from both auditory and visual hallucinations.

CHAPTER 3

TOLERANCE, DEPENDENCE, AND MENTAL HEALTH

*L*ike other drugs, PCP is used regularly by some people and infrequently by others. How often a person takes a drug is an important factor in determining its physical and psychological effect. With frequent use, tolerance to a drug often develops. This means that the user needs ever larger doses to achieve the effects produced previously by a smaller dose. Tolerance may also be experienced as a decrease in the duration of the drug's effects. Users may also develop tolerance to some of the behavioral effects of PCP and not to others.

For example, repeated administration of PCP as a veterinary anesthetic to monkeys resulted in shorter periods of anesthesia after several weeks or months of use. Users of PCP who have a history of long exposure to the drug often report a marked increase in their tolerance. Those who initially smoked two to three PCP "joints" per day may, after regular use, increase the amount they smoke to twice that amount or more. Similar observations of tolerance have been noted in humans who are treated for burns with the related drug ketamine.

To understand the way PCP works on the body it is essential to study tolerance and loss of tolerance in animals. In some studies, frequent administration of PCP has been shown to produce tolerance. Twice as much of the drug became necessary to disrupt behavior that is reinforced by food and water. This suggests that if people use PCP frequently, they will have to double the dose to produce the desired effect. Laboratory studies indicate that the tolerance that develops to PCP from regular use is mainly physiological (physical), rather than behavioral, or learned.

Behavioral tolerance is the name given to the process whereby users learn to compensate for, or to overcome, the disruptive effects that the drug has on normal behavior. The amount of tolerance a user develops depends on the specific behaviors that occur while under the influence of the drug (for example, driving, or performance at school or on the job) and how often those behaviors are practiced while the individual is under the influence of the drug.

A standard test used to distinguish between behavioral and physiological tolerance to a drug is usually conducted with rats. There are two groups of animals. Each day, one group is injected with a drug (such as PCP) *before* they perform a task (such as pushing on a lever for a drink of

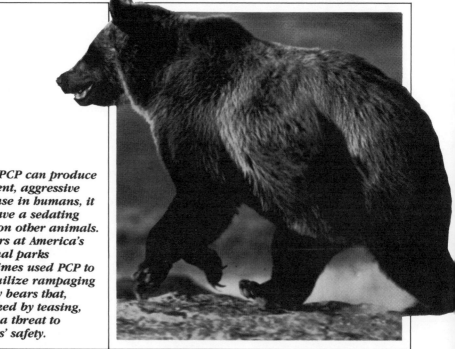

While PCP can produce a violent, aggressive response in humans, it can have a sedating effect on other animals. Rangers at America's national parks sometimes used PCP to tranquilize rampaging grizzly bears that, provoked by teasing, posed a threat to visitors' safety.

water). Thus, they must learn to perform the task while under the influence of the drug. The other group is injected with the same amount of the drug *after* they perform the task. Therefore, both groups have the same repeated exposure to the drug, and the same amount of practice at the task, but the second group does *not* have to perform the task while under the influence of the drug.

After a number of days both groups are injected *before* they perform the task. If they perform equally well, it is likely that physiological changes have contributed to the development of tolerance. If only the group that was injected before the task shows improved behavior, then behavioral tolerance would explain the effect. This is because this group, while under the influence of the drug, had repeated experience with the task and ample time to learn to compen-

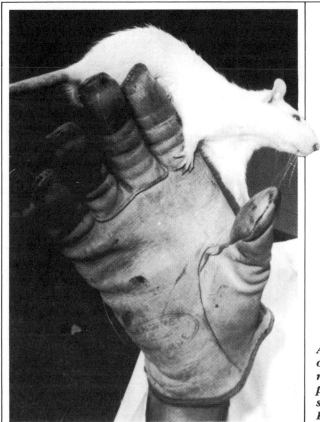

A laboratory rat perches on the gloved hand of a researcher. Rats have proved invaluable in studies on the effects of PCP and other drugs.

sate for the drug's effects. When this experiment was conducted with PCP, both groups performed equally well, suggesting that tolerance was based on physiological factors.

Physiological tolerance is attributed to such factors as heightened sensitivity to the drug at brain receptor sites or increased rate of metabolism and excretion of the drug due to an increase in the production of enzymes. It is important to understand the difference between behavioral and physiological tolerance, since tolerance, especially tolerance that produces potentially irreversible physiological changes, may be related to the development of drug dependence. However, it is likely that to some degree both behavioral and physiological mechanisms play an important role in the development of tolerance to most drugs.

Other laboratory studies with rats showed that within a few days of regular use or nonuse, tolerance can be repeat-

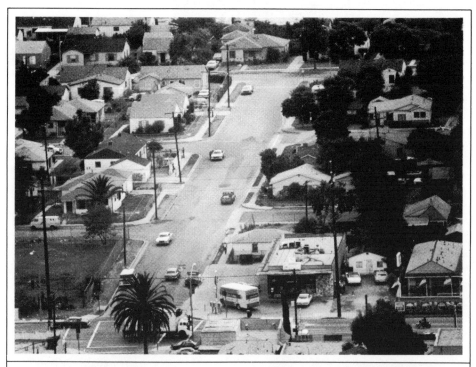

Compton, California, was a quiet, middle-class town until it became the center of a flourishing PCP market in the 1980s. Violence accompanying the drug trade included the fatal shooting of a teenage dealer.

edly acquired and lost. It seems, therefore, that tolerance to PCP is closely related to the frequency with which it is used and is most likely to develop when PCP is used several times each week. When a regular user abruptly stops taking PCP for a period of time, tolerance is rapidly lost. If, after this loss of tolerance, the PCP user were to take the amount he was previously taking, unexpected adverse effects or even an overdose could occur. If complete tolerance had developed and been lost, it is possible that, upon returning to the drug, the user would need only half his previous dose to achieve the level of effect he experienced before.

The development of tolerance manifests itself differently in each subject. In most animal studies, tolerance develops as expected, with a decrease in the effect of a given dose after regular use, yet there are always some animals who show no tolerance at all. Similarly, while most regular PCP users report that tolerance has developed, others do not. Since the variety of forms in which drugs are sold on the street is so great, a user can never know with any accuracy the exact PCP content of the drug he or she has taken. When we add to this the fact that in the street environment the drug is rarely taken at regular intervals, and that the user's performance can never be objectively observed, any attempt to measure human tolerance to PCP becomes extremely difficult.

How Dependence Grows

"Drug dependence" is a term that usually refers to measurable patterns of repeated drug use. The term has become widely accepted by those who study the behavioral action of drugs. According to this definition, all drug use, whether infrequent or continuous, reflects some degree of drug dependence.

Terms previously used to define drug dependence were "drug addiction" and "drug abuse." Psychological dependence was defined as "craving," "satisfaction," "pleasure leading to drug use," or a "drive to repeatedly use drugs to obtain pleasure or avoid discomfort." Another indication of psychological dependence has been said to be a "propensity to relapse to habitual drug use after a long drug-free period." These descriptions are not as useful as the term *drug dependence*, because they are all difficult to measure.

The terms "physical dependence" and "physiological dependence" are used interchangeably. They refer to behavior that occurs when a person stops taking PCP after having taken it for a long time. The disruptions that result are called withdrawal symptoms. Both painful and debilitating, they have been described as resembling a severe case of influenza. Withdrawal symptoms can usually be quickly reversed either by again taking the drug, or by taking a similar drug. While physical dependence is often part of the general picture of drug dependence, it does not always occur. For instance, stopping a marijuana habit may not result in withdrawal symptoms or any signs of physical distress, yet the drug reinforces long sequences of complex behavior leading to renewed use.

Physical dependence can also occur in situations where the individual has not taken the drug voluntarily. For example, a hospital patient may suffer withdrawal symptoms when pain-killing morphine treatments are discontinued. And infants born to drug-dependent mothers can exhibit withdrawal symptoms, indicating that physical dependence has developed.

Withdrawing from PCP

Although physical or physiological dependence on PCP has not yet been extensively documented in studies on people, there is some evidence that withdrawal symptoms occur when a user stops taking the drug. One study in the early 1980s revealed that one-third of 68 regular PCP users tried to find treatment or obtain medication to help them stop taking PCP. When they did stop, they claimed to have experienced symptoms of depression, drug craving, increased appetite, increased need for sleep, and laziness. These symptoms usually lasted from one week to one month after PCP use had been discontinued, corresponding to the amount of time needed to clear PCP from the body.

Infants born to mothers who took PCP throughout their pregnancy experience withdrawal symptoms such as irritability, tremors, hyperresponsiveness, poor feeding, and high-pitched crying. A third of the infants studied were born at least two weeks earlier than babies born to nondrug-dependent mothers, and their birth weights and sizes were less than that of nondrug-dependent babies born two weeks prematurely. (For more information on PCP and pregnancy, see Chapter 4, "The Long-term Effects of PCP.")

The lack of withdrawal symptoms in some adults may be due to the small doses taken. Or symptoms may not have been severe enough to send patients to a medical facility. Also, users may be unable to distinguish the withdrawal symptoms from the behavioral effects of PCP, which can linger for several days or weeks.

In laboratory studies with monkeys who received PCP intravenously—rather than by smoking it or ingesting it orally, the ways that humans normally use the drug—very clear PCP withdrawal symptoms have been observed. An initial report on the effects of terminating continuous intravenous PCP administration in rhesus monkeys revealed a series of symptoms that began four to eight hours after access to the PCP stopped. The reaction peaked at 12 to 16 hours and subsided in 24 to 48 hours. The symptoms included increased

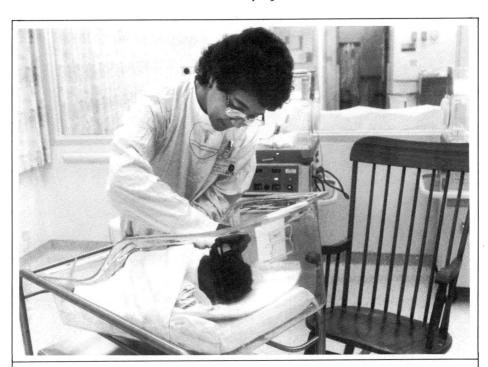

A medical social worker in California attends to the needs of an infant whose mother regularly used PCP during pregnancy. Born "high," such babies may suffer irreversible physical and mental damage.

vocalization, hyperactivity, overly responsive eye movements, vomiting, and diarrhea, though not all symptoms appeared in every monkey. Withdrawal was immediately reversed by an intravenous injection of PCP.

In another study monkeys were trained to press on a lever to receive banana-flavored pellets. At the same time, they received a continuous intravenous dose of PCP. During the first 48 hours after the intravenous infusion was stopped the monkeys exhibited the usual signs of illness, and their rate of pressing the lever for food was low. In fact, the rate became so low that it became necessary to supplement their diet with preferred foods (fruit) to maintain their health. The monkeys did not earn their usual number of banana pellets until nine days after the PCP was stopped. These studies clearly indicate that not only are there painful withdrawal symptoms when animals stop taking PCP, but also more subtle behavioral ones.

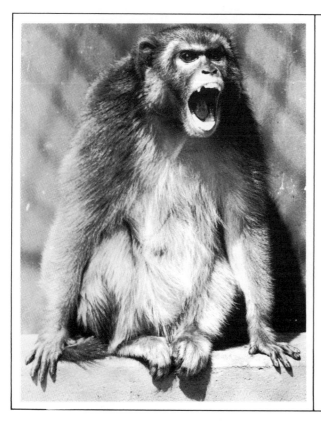

Suddenly deprived of the PCP injections they had been receiving in a laboratory experiment, rhesus monkeys became highly agitated, one indication that they were experiencing withdrawal reactions.

PCP and Mental Health

Since PCP psychosis was first indentified in 1974, there has been considerable interest in comparing the symptoms of PCP psychosis with those experienced by a true psychotic. There has also been an attempt to compare the effects of PCP in psychotic and normal individuals. PCP psychosis, most common in regular PCP users, resembles temporary schizophrenic behavior lasting from one to seven days.

Thought disorders and social withdrawal are symptoms common to both PCP psychosis and schizophrenia. PCP phychosis, however, is not identical to schizophrenia, as PCP use appears to produce a higher incidence of violent, aggressive, threatening, and self-destructive behavior, as well as tension, anxiety, and visual distortion. Those with PCP psychosis also tend to be more independent of their families.

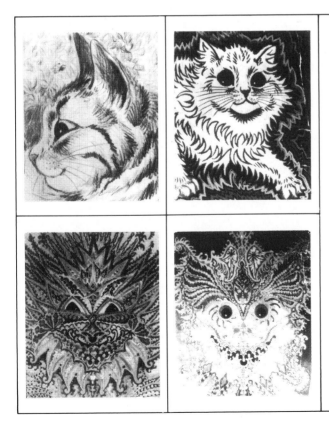

These four pictures were drawn during the course of his illness by a schizophrenic British artist once celebrated for his paintings of cats. People with a history of schizophrenia or other psychotic disorders are prone to mental and visual deterioration similar to that associated with severe PCP psychosis.

A study of 35 people with PCP psychosis who were compared with 11 people with acute schizophrenia found very few differences between the two groups. Among the PCP users there was a greater incidence of trouble with the law, visual hallucinations, and liver disorders.

PCP psychosis has also been compared to the effects of sensory isolation. Research suggests that PCP psychosis is the result of a blockage of sensory input to the brain. It is interesting to note that sensory isolation does not intensify the effects of PCP. Rather it seems to reduce the negative effects of high doses of PCP.

It has also been found that PCP has the ability to intensify the primary symptoms of schizophrenia. In one study, schizophrenics and normal volunteers were given PCP, LSD, and other hallucinogens. Schizophrenics were less affected than the normal volunteers when given LSD or mescaline, and were able to differentiate between the effects of the drugs and the symptoms of their illness. However, PCP intensified their psychotic symptoms. They became more assertive and hostile, and this lasted for as long as six weeks. In normal subjects, PCP produced schizophrenic symptoms which lasted only a few days.

Though it is relatively rare, people who are naturally susceptible to schizophrenia have exhibited psychotic behavior after taking PCP just once. In one such case, a 26-year-old woman with a long history of psychiatric problems, including hospitalization for psychosis, but no history of alcohol or drug abuse, was at a party and shared a joint of "angel dust." After smoking about half the joint, she became paranoid, delusional, and developed both auditory and visual hallucinations. After two days she was admitted to a psychiatric hospital where she remained for over two weeks. Her thought disorder gradually faded, but her depression continued. Eventually, she responded to treatment with antipsychotic drugs.

In the previously mentioned 1980 study of 35 cases of PCP psychosis, six were later hospitalized and diagnosed with acute schizophrenia, though they had had no additional contact with PCP. Two of these patients were finally diagnosed as chronic schizophrenics.

Another study, this time of 40 hospitalized schizophrenics, found that the 26 patients who had previously taken PCP and hallucinogenic drugs had a significantly earlier onset of schizophrenia, earlier admission to the hospital, and earlier diagnosis than the 14 who had not used drugs.

The results of these studies and similar, more recent research into the relationship between PCP psychosis and psychiatric illness raise further questions still to be answered: Does PCP bring about chronic schizophrenia in susceptible individuals? PCP psychosis and schizophrenia might be different terms for the same illness, or do they display similar symptoms of different illnesses? While the explanation for PCP psychosis remains unknown, it is certain that PCP is especially dangerous when taken by schizophrenics or those who have a family history of schizophrenia or other psychotic disorders.

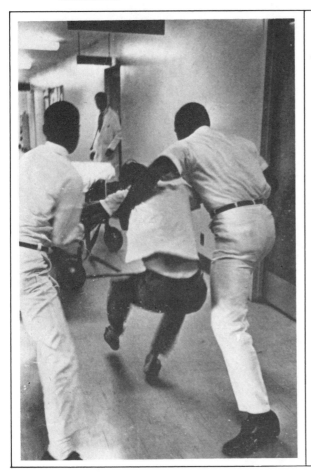

Hospital orderlies struggle with a violent patient suffering from PCP psychosis. When a schizophrenic uses PCP, his or her psychotic symptoms are intensified and the patient may continue to exhibit exaggerated hostility and assertiveness for up to six weeks following the single dosage.

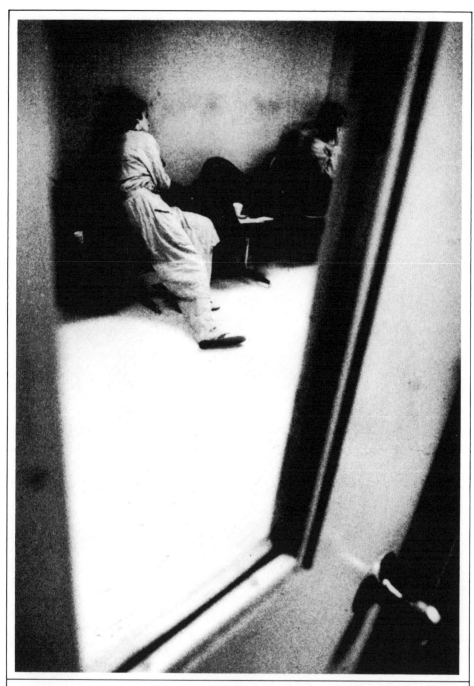

Severe depression is often precipitated by a PCP user's attempt to discontinue use. If this feeling becomes overwhelming, the user may return to the drug, desperately ingest a large dose, and risk overdose.

CHAPTER 4

THE LONG-TERM EFFECTS OF PCP

Because no standardized tests have been given to chronic users, most of the reports on the chronic use of PCP are based on users' perceptions and questionnaire data. However, the data are consistent about the pattern of chronic use and behavioral toxicity.

One study was conducted with 20 chronic PCP users who had taken PCP regularly for six months to five years (an average duration of 27.5 months) before the time of the study. Eight of the users smoked PCP in the form of cigarettes or "joints," while two members of the group "snorted" PCP. It was typically used in two- to three-day bursts or "runs" during which the drug was used continuously and in a social setting where no one slept. A run might be repeated two to four times a month. An average of 10 to 20 PCP cigarettes were smoked each day by each participant, though occasionally one person might smoke many more than 20. The runs were usually followed by one to two days of continuous sleep, from which the subjects awoke disoriented and depressed.

The patterns of chronic PCP use are similar to those of regular amphetamine use. During a period of intense PCP intake, the users tend to eat less, often as little as one meal a day, and in the process lose weight.

Common physical effects noted by this group were constipation, urinary hesitancy, and uncontrollable vertical and horizontal eye movements. Some of them experienced psychological effects such as increased anxiety and nervousness, social withdrawal and isolation, violent and aggressive behavior, paranoid delusions, auditory hallucinations, depression, suicidal and homicidal tendencies, and other personality changes.

One-third of the chronic users reported a gradual change in mood. They believed that PCP had made them more angry, irritable, violent, antisocial, depressed, lonely, or isolated. However, 16% reported positive personality changes. They felt more comfortable, better adjusted to social situations,

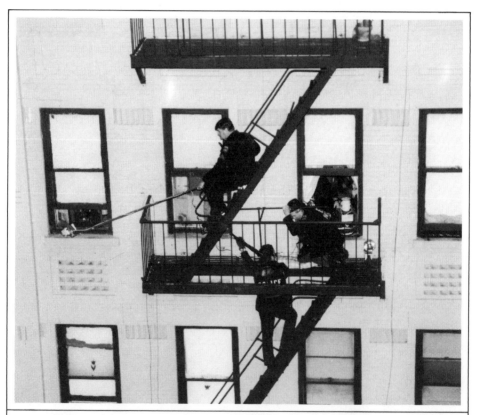

New York City police respond to a distraught man threatening violence and suicide. The unique properties of PCP—increasing drives and reducing inhibitions—often lead to homicidal and suicidal impulses.

more "masculine," and thought they worked better. A number of other psychological effects which first appeared during chronic use persisted for several months to a year after daily use of large doses had stopped. These included periods of disorientation, loss of memory for recent events, persistent slurring of speech, impaired articulation of speech, blockage of speech, and inability to recall appropriate words.

Is PCP Toxic?

Whether chronic PCP use produces lasting changes in personality, biological functions, brain and nerve functions, reproductive functions, and in the health of the user's offspring is a question that continues to be investigated. To date, researchers have found no evidence of permanent damage to the cells and organs of the body from PCP use. In fact,

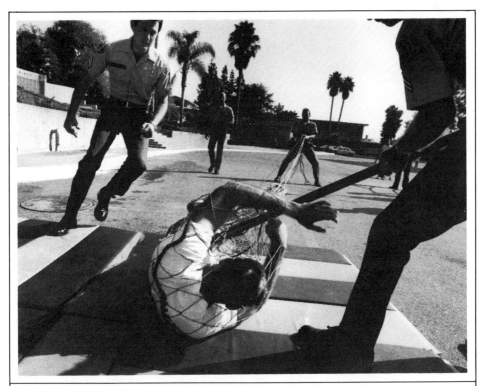

Los Angeles County sheriffs use a net to capture a violent PCP user. Chronic PCP users often experience feelings of superhuman strength and omnipotence. "God is with me and I can move mountains," one user claimed.

during the 1980s scientists studying neurodegenerative diseases (diseases characterized by deterioration of the nervous system) identified what appeared to be helpful properties in PCP that protected the brain from damage during a stroke. However, following up on this research, doctors at the Washington University School of Medicine in St. Louis reported in 1989 that PCP has a toxic effect on brain neurons. Changes in the neurons—cells which are the basic units of nerve tissue—of adult rats were observed after the rats were given relatively low doses of PCP and several related drugs, including ketamine. Although the changes did not increase in severity during long-term administration of the drugs and the effects gradually diminished when the drugs were stopped, scientists believe that these findings "reinforce concern" about the potential risks of using PCP.

New concerns have also been raised about the effects of PCP on the fetuses of pregnant women. In 1989 doctors at the University of California School of Medicine in Los Angeles reported on a study showing that injections of PCP in rats during pregnancy can result in higher levels of the drug in the fetal and neonatal (newborn) brain than in the mother. Their findings suggest that after PCP use is discontinued, PCP disappears more slowly from the brain of the newborn than it does from the brain of the adult, with possible negative consequences for the newborn, including disruption of neurological and behavioral development.

The greatest confirmed danger of PCP use continues to be its behavioral toxicity, or its harmful behavioral effects. While most frequently PCP is initially used in a social setting, individual users soon become isolated and withdrawn. There is a high incidence of divorce, job loss, and disrupted education among chronic PCP users, just as there is among abusers of such drugs as alcohol and marijuana. However, the probability of violent, assaultive, and bizarre behavior is higher in chronic PCP users.

A comparison of chronic and occasional users revealed that the chronic users were more likely to experience violent effects and negative thoughts from a typical PCP experience. They were also more likely to experience elevated mood states. Chronic users showed a greater contrast between their moods before and after PCP use than did occasional users. Chronic PCP users also reported that they felt less sexual, less energetic, and less spirited after emerging from the PCP "high." Whether chronic PCP use permanently changes personality characteristics or whether disproportionately large numbers of individuals with mental disorders are drawn to chronic PCP use are still unanswered questions.

PCP, Depression, and Death

Although the underlying cause of PCP-induced depression is unknown, the evidence suggests that such depression is most frequent among regular users and rarely afflicts those who only occasionally use the drug.

Episodes of depression often follow periods of acute PCP toxicity or PCP psychosis. During this depression, which can last from a few days to several months, there is a high risk of suicide and a high risk of relapse to regular use.

People who stop taking PCP after a long period of use frequently return to it to relieve the depression that is a common withdrawal symptom. In one case a 19-year-old

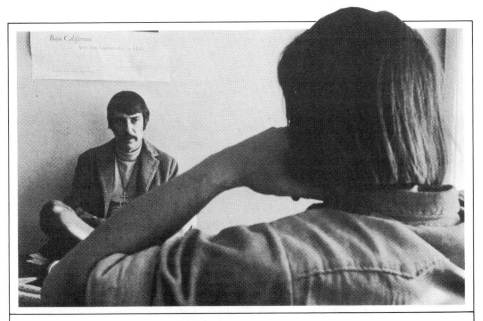

A psychiatrist and his patient discuss PCP-induced depression in the Haight-Ashbury Free Medical Clinic in San Francisco in the late 1960s. PCP first surfaced in this district, once called the "hippie capital" of the United States.

woman who came to a clinic after a PCP overdose described a long history of depression and suicidal thoughts which she was only able to relieve by snorting PCP. However, when she stopped using PCP, the depression which followed was even worse than the one she had experienced before. She stated that she had no intention of stopping PCP use despite her overdose episode. This endless cycle can only be broken by seeking professional help.

Hospitalization is usually required for treatment of PCP-induced depression. This is because on an outpatient basis users fail to regularly attend individual or group therapy sessions or follow their antidepressant drug therapy. In addition, outside the hospital these users continue to take PCP and a variety of other drugs. Further research is needed in order to determine the underlying basis of PCP-induced depression and to develop effective means of therapy.

Although deaths have occurred from overdoses of PCP, more people die from the results of behavior brought about by its use than from the drug's direct effects on the body. Deaths resulting from drowning, accidents, burns, and aggressive behavior have occurred in incidents subsequent to the taking of PCP.

Why PCP Use Persists

PCP's low cost, ease of synthesis, and its ability to substitute for or enhance the effects of other drugs have resulted in high profits and continued use despite its negative consequences. When regular PCP users were questioned about their continued use of PCP, they most frequently answered that they were unable to stop, unwilling to forgo the positive aspects of PCP, and fearful of the pain and depression associated with withdrawal. Indeed, many users who have suffered severe consequences of PCP continue to use it, stating that the bad effects were due to impurities in the drug or to an excessive dose. They also returned to PCP because it was available when no other drug could be found or because they could not afford more expensive drugs.

There have been a number of other possible explanations for the persistence of PCP use. One suggestion is that the users are reinforced by any change in mood, whether positive or negative. Native Hawaiian Job Corps volunteers reported that they used PCP to relieve boredom and to overcome loneliness. Some users claim that they use PCP because it provides a feeling of "nothingness" which is preferable to their own negative feelings. In addition to the withdrawal symptom of depression, chronic users will also admit to occasionally having "bad trips." However, they consider these negative effects a fair price to pay for the possibility of an extraordinary high.

For some, the very unpredictability of having a pleasant experience is its own reward. There is an almost equal chance that the effects will be positive or negative, and this element of chance may appeal to those captivated by risk-taking and the resulting sensations of power and invincibility. In addition, scientific experiments have shown that if a certain behavior is rewarded only some of the time, when the reward is withheld the behavior continues longer than it would if it had been rewarded all of the time. This fact may help to explain why the occasional occurrence of a positive effect amidst many negative effects would cause PCP-using behavior to persist.

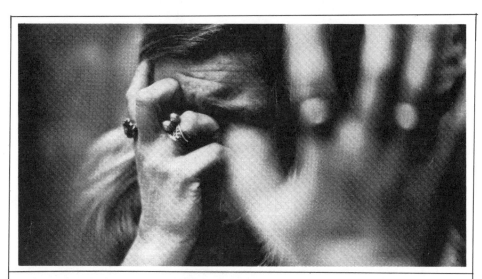

Depending on the individual's personality, mood, and family history of mental illness, the effects of drugs can vary widely. This, in combination with PCP's unpredictability, can produce terrifying, dangerous results.

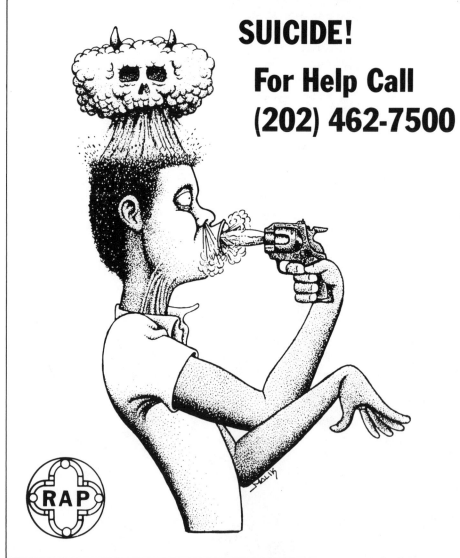

The Regional Addiction Prevention program (RAP), Washington, D.C., circulated this poster in its effort to combat PCP use in the capital's inner city.

CHAPTER 5

THE TREATMENT OF PCP ABUSE

Regardless of whether PCP is snorted, smoked, taken orally, or intravenously, it rapidly leaves the blood, excreting very little into the urine. While some of the drug is metabolized by the liver, since it is highly fat-soluble a large proportion is stored in fatty or brain tissue. Only approximately half of the PCP that is taken leaves the body within three days, which may account for the prolonged effects of overdose leading to coma or PCP psychosis.

When PCP enters the stomach, whether it has been taken orally or secreted from the blood as a result of an intravenous injection or inhalation, very little is absorbed. The contents of the stomach, including PCP, empty into the small intestine where the PCP is reabsorbed into the blood and recirculated in the body.

Because of this characteristic of PCP, right after taking it one would expect the stomach contents to have a high level of PCP. But because of the agitated state of the user at the time he or she is ill enough to require treatment, it is usually impossible to pump the stomach. Tests of the stomach contents would be most useful in determining whether or not a death was related to PCP overdose. However, high drug levels in the stomach would not necessarily indicate that the overdose victim had taken the drug orally. The amount of PCP in the stomach would be high regardless of how the drug was taken because PCP also enters the stomach from the blood.

Except in cases of massive overdose, the amount of PCP detected in the blood and urine is not an accurate indicator of how much PCP the person took because it is highly dependent upon the acidity of the blood, and will also be influenced by what the user has had to drink. Although there are methods for measuring the amount of PCP in the blood and urine, all of them, especially those that pick up trace amounts, have proven to be expensive and time-consuming. In addition, some methods produce false results. Clearly this situation makes it difficult and impractical to obtain reliable measurements of PCP from the body fluids, measurements necessary for proper treatment.

PCP Antidotes

An antidote is a drug or chemical that can be given to reverse the effects of another drug. For example, when the drug Narcan is administered to a person who has overdosed on heroin, the effects are completely reversed and the individual rapidly returns to a normal state. Though there is currently no antidote for PCP, research efforts have yielded some promising results. In 1982 a report announced the discovery of two compounds that blocked the effects of PCP in rats. Researchers at the University of Arizona reported in 1987 on experiments in which dogs were treated with PCP-derived antigens (substances capable of stimulating a response from the body's immune system) which reversed the toxic effects of PCP after the drug had been administered in small doses. Further experiments are continuing with other animals to reverse the toxicity of higher doses.

Currently the standard treatment for PCP "intoxication" in hospital emergency rooms is either ammonium chloride tablets or cranberry juice with vitamin C. These "flush out" the system, drawing out PCP from body tissues and putting it back into the bloodstream where it is eventually eliminated. Although these substances are not, strictly speaking, antidotes, since they are not known to reverse any effects the drug has already had on cells and organs, they at least prevent possible further damage by hastening PCP's elimination from the body. Until a safe and well-tested antidote is found, treatment for PCP abuse will continue to consist chiefly of managing symptoms and vital signs.

Table 4

Indications of Acute PCP Intoxication Within an hour of use of PCP or a similar drug at least two of the following symptoms would appear:	
PHYSICAL	PSYCHOLOGICAL
Rapid vertical or horizontal eye movement Increased blood pressure and heart rate Numbness or low responsiveness to pain Loss of coordination Speech difficulty	Euphoria Agitation Anxiety Emotional swings Grandiose thoughts Sensation of slowed time Feeling or sensation in one part of the body produced by stimulation of another part

Treating Acute PCP Intoxication

The diagnosis of acute PCP intoxication is made if the patient does not exhibit any of the signs and symptoms of a psychotic reaction (e.g., violence and self-destructive behavior), or the symptoms of overdose, such as severe sedation or coma. Thus it seems that acute PCP intoxication is diagnosed by what it is not. The complete list of symptoms, taken from a medical diagnostic manual, it shown in Table 4.

The first step in treatment is usually to detoxify the patient by giving him either ammonium chloride pills or cranberry juice with vitamin C (see above). Acute PCP intoxication lasts between six and eight hours, but signs of improvement usually appear within two to four hours. Since the anesthetic effects of the drug greatly reduce the pain associated with serious injury, the patient has to be prevented from injuring himself. This is accomplished by secluding the intoxicated user in a nonstimulating environment where contact with other people is minimal. After recovering from intoxication, the user is closely monitored for PCP psychosis, depression, and/or suicidal thoughts. Physical restraints may be necessary, and tranquilizers such as Valium have been used successfully to control agitation. A severe psychosis may be treated with Haldol, an antipsychotic prescription drug. Confirming the diagnosis of PCP intoxication is done by searching through the patient's personal belongings, questioning anyone who may have been present during the taking of the drug, and, if possible, by testing the patient's stomach contents and bodily fluids.

Diagnosing and Treating PCP Overdose

There are several problems involved in determining whether or not a person has taken an overdose of PCP. It may be impossible to obtain the victim's history either because the overdose victim is in a coma, or he is suffering from amnesia (another symptom of overdose) and does not remember what drug he has taken. In some cases the patient only knows the drug's street name, which is often a poor indicator of the drug's actual contents.

As previously mentioned, urine and blood tests which measure PCP content in the body are generally not reliable both because of the delays involved in testing and receiving laboratory results and because of the speed with which PCP leaves these fluids. The behavioral and physical symptoms which would support a diagnosis of PCP overdose are:

Prolonged coma (1 day to 2 weeks)
Eyes usually closed but may remain open
Elevated blood pressure
Muscle rigidity
Profuse sweating
Excessive salivation
Convulsions
Rapid horizontal and vertical eye movement
Repetitive motor movements
Decreased response of the cornea to light (corneal reflex)
Decreased gagging response when the back of the throat is stimulated (gag reflex)
Absence of mild sensation
Fever, flushing

While the use of a respirator is rarely necessary for patients suffering from the effects of PCP overdose, a combination of PCP with alcohol, sedatives, or opiates greatly increases the likelihood of respiratory complications.

The initial phase of PCP overdose treatment consists of basic life-support measures including maintenance and monitoring of body fluids, pulse, and respiration. The drug may be removed from the body by pumping out the contents of the stomach, or diuretics may be administered to increase the production and flow of urine to flush out the PCP.

Coming out of the coma, the patient may exhibit many signs of PCP psychosis. Putting the patient in an isolated environment will help reduce violence, excitability, anxiety, paranoia, and irritability. During this stage, patients often become unmanageable, and restraints and/or tranquilizers may be necessary. Life-support measures are still essential during this phase, and stomach suctioning is usually continued for at least three days following recovery from coma. Also, since during this recovery phase some patients become confused and even suicidal, psychiatric care may be necessary.

Diagnosing and Treating PCP Psychosis

In the late 1970s PCP psychosis was a leading cause of admissions to psychiatric wards. However, due to its remarkable similarity to schizophrenia, it was often misdiagnosed.

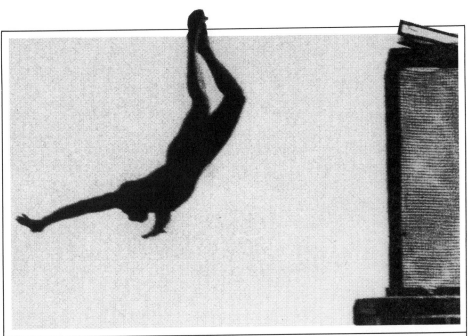

A New York City youth diving to his death. Chronic PCP use can lead to hopelessness and depression. Before committing suicide one PCP user wrote, "My suicide is a must. I am full of anxiety. Depression is too much."

Table 5

Three Stages of PCP Psychosis		
AGITATED PHASE (3 to 5 days)	MIXED PHASE (3 to 5 days)	RESOLUTION PHASE (3 to 5 days)
Sleepiness Loss of appetite Restlessness Hyperactive behavior Auditory hallucinations Violent, aggressive behavior Thought disorders Paranoia Delusions	Some improvement Confusion Thought disorders Hallucinations Blocking of speech Paranoia	Return to previous personality Improved memory Decreased paranoia Improvement of thought disorders

It is also difficult to diagnose because PCP psychosis may occur a week or more after the drug is absent from the body fluids. PCP psychosis is usually considered if the patient has a history of drug abuse or enters the hospital exhibiting schizophrenic or other bizarre behaviors.

There are at least three different phases of PCP psychosis, each of which requires a somewhat different treatment (see Table 5).

During the *agitated phase* treatment consists of hospitalization in a psychiatric ward, with seclusion in a room that offers minimal stimulation. Treatment with antipsychotic drugs such as Haldol may be used to reduce the agitation and hyperactivity, although PCP psychosis does not respond as well or as readily as does schizophrenia. The minor tranquilizers such as Valium are not useful in treating PCP psychosis and may actually increase the level of agitation.

Another treatment, acidification of the urine, allows PCP to be passed through the small intestine to the liver and kidneys from where it is excreted. Since at this point the patient's cooperation may be difficult to obtain, it may be necessary to wait for the severe psychotic symptoms to subside before beginning the process, which is usually continued for at least three days after all signs of psychosis have disappeared.

The *mixed phase* usually begins about five days after the patient seeks treatment, or after three days if urine acidification has been performed. This phase contains periodic recurrences of the agitated phase, including violence and paranoia, which make the patient unpredictable and dangerous.

Treatment during the mixed phase consists of reducing the amount of seclusion and observing the patient carefully to determine whether his or her behavior is under control. If not, further isolation may be needed. Psychotic behavior is modified by continuing medication and involving the patient in group therapy. Finally, if the patient was too unmanageable during the initial phase, urine acidification is now begun.

During the *resolution phase* patients are usually followed on an outpatient basis. Upon discharge, almost half of the patients return to PCP use within two weeks, and these patients will be especially prone to another psychotic episode. Improvement tends to be slower in those who did not undergo acidification or in those who are susceptible to schizophrenia. For these patients antipsychotic medication must be continued for a longer period of time.

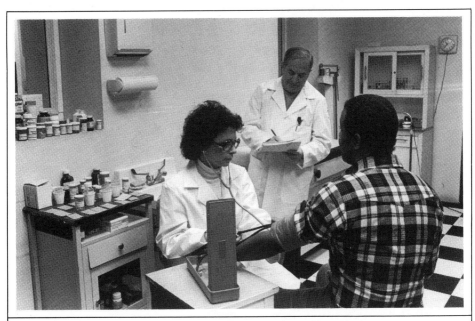

A patient's blood pressure is measured at Phoenix House, a New York City drug rehabilitation center. Elevated blood pressure and rapid eye movements occur simultaneously in cases of PCP intoxication.

Long-Term Treatment of Chronic PCP Abuse

Chronic PCP abuse is characterized by three main factors:
1. A pattern of pathological use; intoxication throughout the day; episodes of PCP delirium or mental disorder.
2. Impairment of social or occupational functioning due to PCP abuse: fights, loss of friends, absence from work, loss of job, or legal difficulties.
3. Duration of disturbance of at least one month.

Chronic PCP abuse resembles the abuse of other drugs, and PCP users tend to have personality characteristics and life-styles similar to those of other drug users. Therefore, the methods of treatment for chronic PCP users are similar to those used to treat users of other drugs. However, some chronic PCP users do not respond well to standard treat-

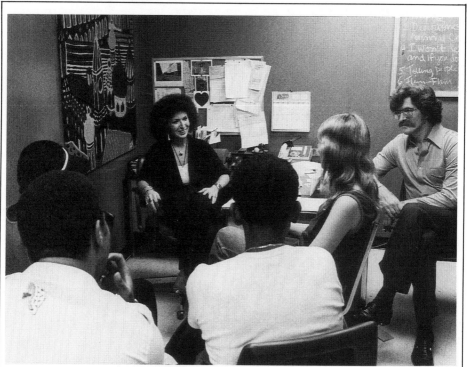

Group therapy is an integral part of the treatment of PCP abuse. While confrontational sessions are potentially hazardous due to clients' unpredictable behavior, small supportive groups are effective.

ment procedures because their judgments and thought processes are impaired.

Patients severely impaired by the long-term effects of PCP would not benefit from a comprehensive treatment plan. In such cases it is often necessary to either postpone long-term treatment until the psychological effects of the drug have subsided or choose a simpler, less demanding plan to reduce irritability and agitation in the patient. Participation in a simple therapy program is useful for these patients.

If the chronic PCP user is relatively unimpaired, an individual treatment plan, such as the one described below, would be employed. Actual treatment plans are often much less comprehensive than this ideal plan, and there have been few formal evaluations of these programs.

Features of a Treatment Plan for PCP Abusers

1. PCP abuse is treated as a primary disorder and not secondary to another problem.

2. The patient is informed that a program is essential and that it consists of many elements.

3. There is an understanding that the program is long term (1–2 years).

4. A crucial feature of the program is change, affecting family interactions, friends, attitudes, and environment.

5. Formal psychiatric assessment and family history are necessary. Drug abusers generally have higher rates of depressive disorders, and PCP users in particular are more likely to show evidence of schizophrenia.

6. The treatment should involve family support.

7. Frequent monitoring of urine and blood to allow for early detection of the use of PCP or other drugs.

8. A community-based, drug-free program to give needed support.

9. Regular appointments with a therapist and periodic contact with the family are essential.

10. A recovering PCP user should be encouraged to serve as a role model for another patient.

11. General health measures such as diet and exercise patterns should be closely monitored.

12. The PCP user should be educated about the effects of PCP and other drugs.

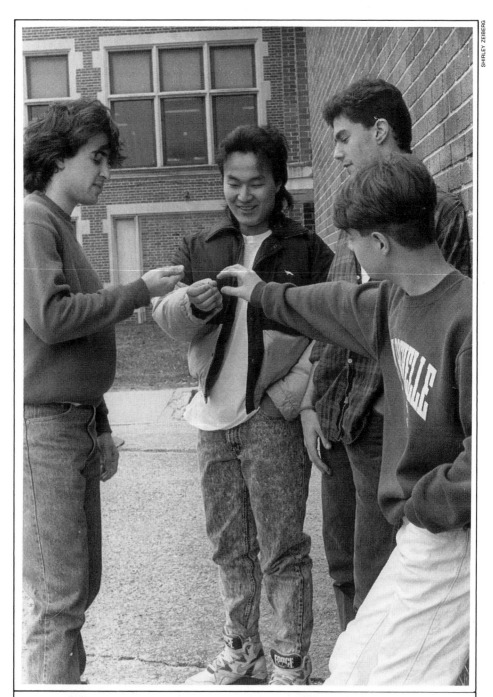

Many teenagers' first use of PCP occurs within the context of smoking marijuana with a small group of friends. Solitary use of PCP often represents the beginning of serious interpersonal problems.

CHAPTER 6

WHO USES PCP?

*T*here are several factors specific to PCP that have prohibited an accurate study of both the cause and spread of its use, and the trends in its use since its introduction as a street drug in 1967. Before 1979 PCP was included in the general class of hallucinogens on most national drug surveys and questions specifically concerned with PCP did not appear during this time, which represented the peak period of widespread abuse of psychoactive drugs. Thus, most of PCP's early statistical history went unrecorded.

The records that were kept almost certainly underestimated PCP use since the drug was often sold as another substance and users were often unaware that they were taking PCP. Users' reports are highly questionable because of the PCP-induced amnesia in combination with PCP's many other effects. Records taken from emergency rooms or treatment facilities were also likely to be unreliable for three reasons: overdose and other adverse effects tended to occur in new users who may have believed they were taking other drugs; many hospitals did not then routinely test for PCP, or if testing was done results were inaccurate; and an acute toxic psychotic episode resulting from PCP abuse was often misdiagnosed as a schizophrenic episode, which meant that PCP screening (if done at all) occurred too late.

Researchers can be encouraged by the fact that these problems have been largely resolved and medical personnel are becoming more knowledgeable about PCP. Today there are several national studies that regularly monitor PCP use and make public reports of their findings.

Sources of Information

The oldest ongoing study of nonprescription drug use in the United States began in 1971 and is called the National Household Survey. Originally established by the National Commission on Marijuana and Drug Abuse to monitor the growing problem of drug abuse, the survey, done at intervals of several years, has been sponsored by the National Institute on Drug Abuse (NIDA) since 1974. The most recent National Household Survey was conducted in 1988; a summary of its findings is included in Appendix I, "Population Estimates of Lifetime and Current Nonmedical Drug Use, 1988." The survey covers the population aged 12 and older living in households in the contiguous United States. Three major age groups are covered: youth, ages 12–17; young adults, ages 18–25; and older adults, age 26 and over. However, while the survey currently monitors the use of thirteen different substances, PCP is included in the category "Hallucinogens" rather than being listed separately.

Another source of nonmedical drug use information is DAWN, the Drug Abuse Warning Network, mentioned briefly in Chapter 1. Established by the U.S. government in the mid-1970s under the sponsorship of NIDA, DAWN is an annual data-collection system that focuses on the involvement of drugs in both hospital emergency room (ER) admissions and medical examiner (ME) autopsy reports in metropolitan areas across the country. Appendixes II and III, drawn from the 1988 DAWN annual report, list drugs mentioned most frequently in ER and ME reports respectively during that year. In 1988 PCP ranked fifth in emergency room mentions and fifteenth in medical examiner reports. The demographic data for PCP emergency room patients in the 1988 DAWN report show that the majority are black (57%), male (75%), and 20–29 years of age (56%). Data on PCP-related deaths show similar distributions for gender (84% male) and age (47% were 20–29 years old). Forty-five percent of those who died were black, 25% white, and 15% Hispanic. When looking at the DAWN data, however, it should be kept in mind that DAWN collects information only from 26 major metropolitan areas; the extent of use of PCP or any other drug in smaller cities or in rural areas is thus not reflected in the DAWN reports.

A third source of drug use information is the National High School Senior Survey, "Monitoring the Future," conducted annually since 1975 for NIDA by the University of Michigan Institute for Social Research. Every year a representative sample of seniors from public and private secondary

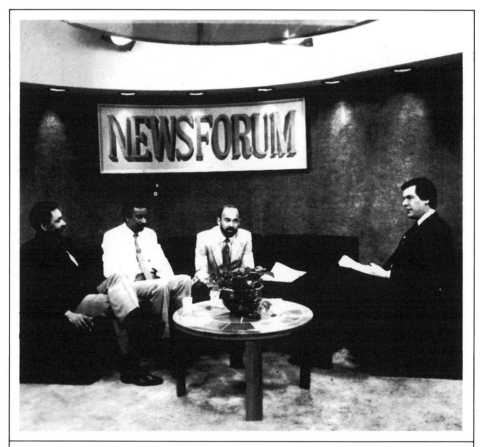

Leaders of RAP explain their antidrug campaign on television. Encouraging community participation and using a family-like environment for residents, RAP struggles to curb the PCP epidemic.

schools is questioned about lifetime, recent (previous year), and current (previous month) drug use. Appendix IV, "National High School Senior Survey, 1975–1989," reports 21 categories of lifetime drug use. Since 1979, PCP use has been a separate category under hallucinogens. In that year, almost 13% of high school seniors reported that they had tried PCP at least once. Afterwards, the percentage of lifetime PCP use declined each year, to a low of 2.9% in 1988. However, in 1989 PCP use was again up: 3.9% of seniors reported they had tried PCP at least once. The survey also showed that 1.4% of seniors had used PCP within the previous month, an increase of more than a percentage point from the 1988 data;

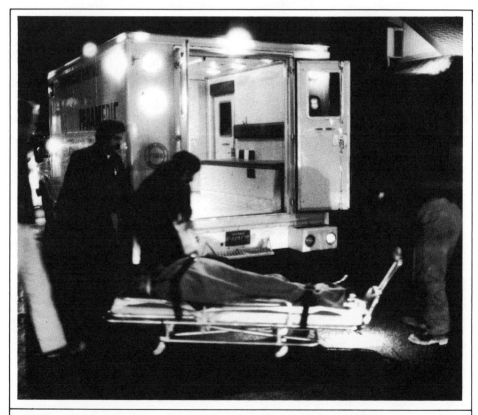

California paramedics remove the body of a teenage victim of PCP overdose. In 1975 DAWN reported 22 PCP-related deaths in the United States; by 1988 this figure had risen to 209.

Table 6

Attitudes of High School Seniors Toward PCP Abuse			
Q: *How much do you think people risk harming themselves (physically or in other ways) if they try PCP once or twice?*	Class of 1987	Class of 1988	Class of 1989
Percentage saying "great risk":	55.6	58.8	56.6
Q: *How many of your friends would you estimate take PCP?*			
Percentage saying none:	84.5	86.5	85.3
Percentage saying most or all:	1.1	0.8	1.2
Q: *How difficult do you think it would be for you to get PCP if you wanted some?*			
Percentage saying "fairly easy" or "very easy":	22.8	24.9	28.9

Source: National Institute on Drug Abuse, National High School Senior Survey: "Monitoring the Future," 1989

0.2% reported being daily PCP users, a slight increase over 1988.

In addition to asking students about drug use, the annual National High School Senior Survey also measures attitudes toward drugs. Table 6, "Attitudes of High School Seniors Toward PCP Abuse," shows no dramatic changes during the three years (1987–89) that PCP has been a separate category in the entire attitudes survey. What may be most significant is that the perceived ability to obtain PCP "fairly easily" or "very easily" increased in 1988 and again—by four percentage points—in 1989. Almost 29% of seniors reported that PCP was available to them. It is also interesting—and of concern—to note that only a little more than half of the seniors perceived a "great risk" in trying PCP once or twice, despite the well-publicized unpredictable nature of the drug.

Trends in PCP Use

During the various "waves" of PCP use since its introduction as a street drug in 1967, different segments of the population have been identified as its primary users: First, so-called hippies seeking a mind-altering experience similar to that induced by LSD; then, teenagers looking for a "high" more powerful than marijuana but easier to obtain than heroin; and in the 1980s, inner city residents of low socioeconomic status and limited education, who chose PCP because of its low cost but would have preferred cocaine if they had been able to afford it. This does not mean, of course, that PCP use in any given year or decade was confined exclusively to a particular group. During the more than 20 years of its street life PCP has probably had a circulation as varied as any of the abused drugs studied by NIDA. Even in Washington, D.C., which has the distinction of being the current "PCP capital" there are middle-class users.

However, stories about bad "trips"—psychotic episodes that have led to murder, coma, or the user's own death—have probably been a significant factor in limiting PCP's use among the middle-class and generally better educated population. The lack of a guarantee that the drug will produce a predictably pleasurable effect has probably been another deterrent among the same group of people. The growth during the 1980s of cocaine as the drug of choice for the middle class pushed PCP further into the background as an option for this group, but among the inner-city poor, who found cocaine priced beyond their means, PCP offered the possibility of pleasure for a very low price.

Studies of chronic PCP users over the years have shown that they generally turn to the drug for the same reasons that

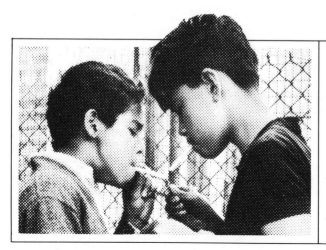

Youngsters who experiment with drugs can never be sure of what they are ingesting. Street drugs sold as THC (the active ingredient in marijuana), mescaline, cocaine, and psilocybin have been analyzed and found to contain high percentages of PCP.

people turn to any mind-altering substance: they are curious, they want to "fit in," and they want to escape from their present situation. PCP offers a bonus, however, particularly to those who feel poor, alienated from society, and incapable of changing their lives: It can produce feelings of power and invulnerability, and the appearance of superhuman strength. The anesthetic effects of PCP reportedly eliminate any sensations of pain in its users, who will fight to the death any would-be subduers. A PCP user experiencing a psychosis can be a very dangerous person indeed.

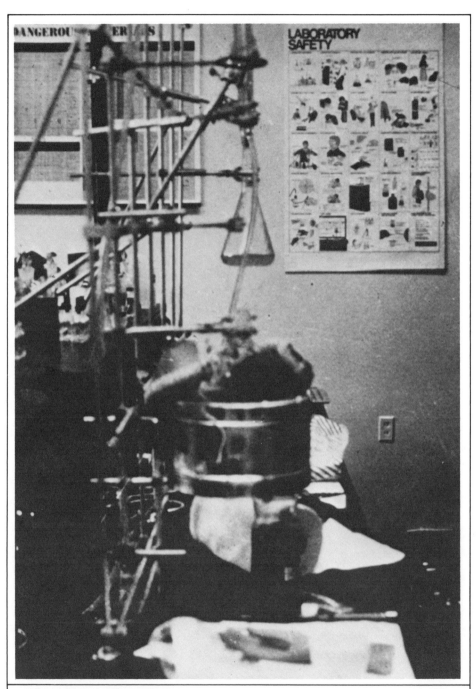

PCP is frequently manufactured in home laboratories similar to this one. Although PCP synthesis is known as "cooking," the three-stage, 18-hour chemical process actually requires no heat.

CHAPTER 7

ECONOMIC AND LEGAL STATUS OF PCP

*T*he widespread availability and low cost of PCP have been major reasons for its continued use. The chemicals needed to make PCP can be easily obtained from chemical supply companies, and an individual with some knowledge of chemistry can synthesize PCP in a kitchen, basement, or garage. Raids on illegal laboratories have yielded up to $25 million worth of PCP. In 1987 a single seizure in Washington, D.C., yielded more than 2 gallons of liquid PCP, ultimately worth about $12 million.

Today most liquid PCP—the most common form of the drug—is manufactured in illegal laboratories in and around Los Angeles. Additional supplies of the liquid come from the New Jersey-Philadelphia region. Washington, D.C., is the hub of East Coast distribution to other cities such as Baltimore, where there is a high demand. Huge profits can be made from selling PCP, a lucrative business in the District of Columbia. About $500 worth of chemicals make one gallon of PCP, which can then be sold to a distributor for $15,000. Distributors sell the PCP in 1-ounce amounts—often in vanilla extract bottles—for between $275 and $300 each to street dealers. A dealer who buys the 1-ounce bottle uses it to treat plant material—marijuana, parsley, oregano, or mint, most commonly—and sells this material on the street in 4–5 ounce tins for \$10–\$15 per tin. Each vanilla extract bottle holds enough PCP to treat about 84 tins.

Thus, despite the great health risks to the eventual users, the possibility of making large amounts of money makes PCP attractive to both dealers and amateur chemists.

PCP, Crime, and the Law

Drugs are scheduled by the federal government depending upon how likely they are to be abused, how likely they are to produce dependence, and whether or not there is a medical use. For instance, a Schedule I drug is not approved for human use, has a good chance of being abused, and requires licensing with the government for research with animals. In contrast, Schedule IV drugs are not likely to be abused and are more easily obtained, such as through a doctor's prescription.

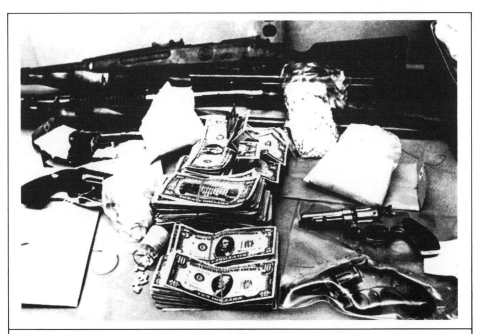

A Washington, D.C., police exhibit of weapons, cash, and drugs seized during a raid on a local dealer. A convicted PCP manufacturer and seller may be sentenced to more than five years in prison.

Since 1978 PCP has been classified as a Schedule II drug under the Comprehensive Drug Abuse Prevention and Control Act of 1970. A drug is classified under Schedule II if there is a high rate of associated abuse, if it has the potential to produce dependence, and if there is an accepted medical use. While there is no accepted medical use for PCP, it can be used for animal anesthesia. However, because of the high rate of illicit PCP use by people in the late 1970s, drug companies ceased making it for animals. Technically, since it now has no medical use, it could be reclassified as a Schedule I drug, but this has not been done. However, many of the drugs that are similar to PCP (e.g., phencyclohexylamine) and its analogs (e.g., PCE, TCP, PCC) are now Schedule I controlled substances.

The penalties for possession, manufacture, and sale of PCP depend upon whether the arrest was made by the DEA (a federal agency) or by a local law enforcement agency. Also, the specific details of each case determine whether an individual is to be tried in federal or local court.

Penalties also vary greatly depending upon the laws of the city or state where a nonfederal case is tried. In general,

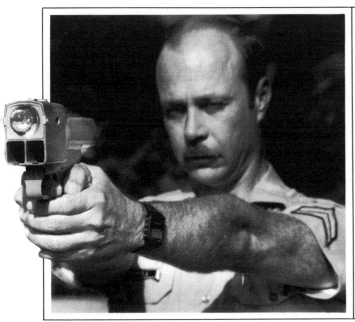

A Los Angeles County deputy sheriff demonstrates the Taser gun, one of the few nonlethal weapons that police officers consider effective against violent PCP users. The Taser fires two darts into its target, followed by an electric shock strong enough to render most people temporarily helpless.

possession of up to one gram of PCP for personal use is considered a misdemeanor, and the DEA is not often involved in these arrests.

Manufacture, sales to several individuals, and possession when arrest takes place can result in a charge of a felony, on several counts. In federal court a first offense can bring a minimum ten-year prison sentence and a fine of up to $4 million. Repeat offenders can be sentenced to 20 years to life in prison, and be fined up to $8 million.

With the possible exception of alcohol, PCP, especially when chronically used, is more closely associated than other drugs with bizarre, unpredictable, and aggressive behavior that may lead to the injury or death of others. However, the actual proportion of PCP-related homicides is low.

In cases of PCP-related murder, defendants have pleaded not guilty by reason of diminished capacity or insanity (drug-induced psychosis). Psychiatrists have studied the diminished-capacity defense with respect to PCP and concluded that PCP interferes with the mental processes essential for forming the intent to act criminally. They claim that not only does PCP alter consciousness and prevent the user

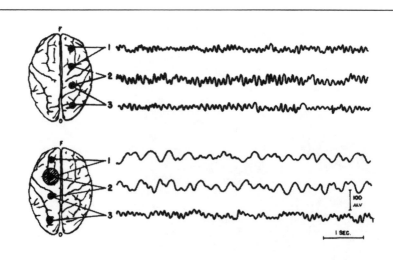

Normal (above) and abnormal brain waves. Lawyers defending clients charged with PCP-related crimes sometimes cite drug-induced brain abnormalities to support pleas based on "diminished capacity."

from responding appropriately to his environment and situation, but it also creates a confusion which alters the meaning of an act or its consequences. Finally, PCP-induced involuntary behavior may prevent intelligent choices of action, and also interfere with goal-directed activity, thus preventing organized physical movements.

The diminished-capacity defense is usually conducted in court by the testimony of an expert witness (usually a psychiatrist who specializes in psychopharmacology). The expert forms an opinion of the defendant's capacity based on findings from physical examinations, recordings of changes in brain waves (EEGs), and in-depth interviewing and testing of the defendant and witnesses.

When this evidence is admitted into court, it is entered as an opinion, not as a scientific fact. Diminished-capacity defenses are not often successful, being more difficult to prove than insanity defenses, which themselves are successful only two-thirds of the time.

Even if the diminished capacity defense is successful, the defendant will be given a reduced sentence and committed to prison. Unlike a successful insanity defense, the defendant would probably not receive treatment for drug abuse or mental health problems at a state mental health facility. If the prison sentence is short, as it may be in the case of voluntary manslaughter with absence of malice due to diminished capacity, it is possible that once back in society other violent acts will be committed by patients suffering from untreated PCP psychosis.

Appendix I

POPULATION ESTIMATES OF LIFETIME AND CURRENT NONMEDICAL DRUG USE, 1988

	12-17 years (pop. 20,250,000)			18-25 years (pop. 29,688,000)		
	%	Ever Used	% Current User	%	Ever Used	% Current User
Marijuana & Hashish	17	3,516,000	6 1,296,000	56	16,741,000	16 4,594,000
Hallucinogens	3	704,000	1 168,000	14	4,093,000	2 569,000
Inhalants	9	1,774,000	2 410,000	12	3,707,000	2 514,000
Cocaine	3	683,000	1 225,000	20	5,858,000	5 1,323,000
Crack	1	188,000	+ +	3	1,000,000	1 249,000
Heroin	1	118,000	+ +	+	+	+ +
Stimulants*	4	852,000	1 245,000	1	3,366,000	2 718,000
Sedatives	2	475,000	1 1 23,000	6	1,633,000	1 265,000
Tranquilizers	2	413,000	+ +	8	2,319,000	1 307,000
Analgesics	4	840,000	1 182,000	9	2,798,000	1 440,000
Alcohol	50	10,161,000	25 5,097,000	90	26,807,000	65 19,392,000
Cigarettes	42	8,564,000	12 2,389,000	75	22,251,000	35 10,447,000
Smokeless Tobacco	15	3,021,000	4 722,000	24	6,971,000	6 1,855,000

* Amphetamines and related substances
+ Amounts of less than .5% are not listed
 Terms: Ever Used: used at least once in a person's lifetime.
  Current User: used at least once in the 30 days prior to the survey.

Source: National Institute on Drug Abuse, August 1989

POPULATION ESTIMATES OF LIFETIME AND CURRENT NONMEDICAL DRUG USE, 1988

26+ years (pop. 148,409,000)				TOTAL (pop. 198,347,000)			
%	Ever Used	%	Current User	%	Ever Used	%	Current User
31	45,491,000	4	5,727,000	33	65,748,000	6	11,616,000
7	9,810,000	+	+	7	4,607,000	+	+
4	5,781,000	+	+	6	1,262,000	1	1,223,000
10	14,631,000	1	1,375,000	11	21,171,000	2	2,923,000
+	+	+	+	1	2,483,000	+	484,000
1	1,686,000	+	+	1	1,907,000	+	+
7	9,850,000	1	791,000	7	4,068,000	1	1,755,000
3	4,867,000	+	+	4	6,975,000	+	+
5	6,750,000	1	822,000	5	9,482,000	1	1,174,000
5	6,619,000	+	+	5	10,257,000	1	1,151,000
89	131,530,000	55	81,356,000	85	168,498,000	53	105,845,000
80	118,191,000	30	44,284,000	75	149,005,000	29	57,121,000
13	19,475,000	3	4,497,000	15	29,467,000	4	7,073,000

Appendix II

DRUGS MENTIONED MOST FREQUENTLY BY HOSPITAL EMERGENCY ROOMS, 1988

	Drug name	Number of mentions by emergency rooms	Percent of total number of mentions
1	Cocaine	62,141	38.80
2	Alcohol-in-combination	46,588	29.09
3	Heroin/Morphine	20,599	12.86
4	Marijuana/Hashish	10,722	6.69
5	PCP/PCP Combinations	8,403	5.25
6	Acetaminophen	6,426	4.01
7	Diazepam	6,082	3.80
8	Aspirin	5,544	3.46
9	Ibuprofen	3,878	2.42
10	Alprazolam	3,846	2.40
11	Methamphetamine/Speed	3,030	1.89
12	Acetaminophen W Codeine	2,457	1.53
13	Amitriptyline	1,960	1.22
14	D.T.C. Sleep Aids	1,820	1.14
15	Methadone	1,715	1.07
16	Triazolam	1,640	1.02
17	Diphenhydramine	1,574	0.98
18	D-Propoxyphene	1,563	0.98
19	Hydantoin	1,442	0.90
20	Lorazepam	1,345	0.84
21	LSD	1,317	0.82
22	Amphetamine	1,316	0.82
23	Phenobarbital	1,223	0.76
24	Oxycodone	1,192	0.74
25	Imipramine	1,064	0.66

Source: Drug Abuse Warning Network (DAWN), Annual Data 1988

Appendix III

DRUGS MENTIONED MOST FREQUENTLY BY MEDICAL EXAMINERS
(IN AUTOPSY REPORTS), 1988

	Drug name	Number of mentions in autopsy reports	Percent of total number of drug mentions
1	Cocaine	3,308	48.96
2	Alcohol-in-combination	2,596	38.43
3	Heroin/Morphine	2,480	36.71
4	Codeine	689	10.20
5	Diazepam	464	6.87
6	Methadone	447	6.62
7	Amitriptyline	402	5.95
8	Nortriptyline	328	4.85
9	Lidocaine	306	4.53
10	Acetaminophen	293	4.34
11	D-Propoxyphene	271	4.01
12	Marijuana/Hashish	263	3.89
13	Quinine	224	3.32
14	Unspec Benzodiazepine	222	3.29
15	PCP/PCP Combinations	209	3.09
16	Diphenhydramine	192	2.84
17	Phenobarbital	183	2.71
18	Desipramine	177	2.62
19	Methamphetamine/Speed	161	2.38
20	Doxepin	152	2.25
21	Aspirin	138	2.04
22	Imipramine	137	2.03
23	Hydantoin	98	1.45
24	Amphetamine	87	1.29
25	Chlordiazepoxide	76	1.12

Source: Drug Abuse Warning Network (DAWN), <u>Annual Data 1988</u>

Appendix IV

NATIONAL HIGH SCHOOL SENIOR SURVEY, 1975-1989

	High School Senior Survey Trends in Lifetime Prevalence Percent Who Ever Used				
	Class of 1975	Class of 1976	Class of 1977	Class of 1978	Class of 1979
Marijuana/Hashish	47.3	52.8	56.4	59.2	60.4
Inhalants	NA	10.3	11.1	12.0	12.7
Inhalants Adjusted	NA	NA	NA	NA	18.2
Amyl & Butyl Nitrites	NA	NA	NA	NA	11.1
Hallucinogens	16.3	15.1	13.9	14.3	14.1
Hallucinogens Adjusted	NA	NA	NA	NA	17.7
LSD	11.3	11.0	9.8	9.7	9.5
PCP	NA	NA	NA	NA	12.8
Cocaine	9.0	9.7	10.8	12.9	15.4
Crack	NA	NA	NA	NA	NA
Other cocaine	NA	NA	NA	NA	NA
Heroin	2.2	1.8	1.8	1.6	1.1
Other Opiates*	9.0	9.6	10.3	9.9	10.1
Stimulants*	22.3	22.6	23.0	22.9	24.2
Stimulants Adjusted*	NA	NA	NA	NA	NA
Sedatives*	18.2	17.7	17.4	16.0	14.6
Barbiturates*	16.9	16.2	15.6	13.7	11.8
Methaqualone*	8.1	7.8	8.5	7.9	8.3
Tranquilizers*	17.0	16.8	18.0	17.0	16.3
Alcohol	90.4	91.9	92.5	93.1	93.0
Cigarettes	73.6	75.4	75.7	75.3	74.0

Stimulants adjusted to exclude inappropriate reporting of nonprescription stimulants; stimulants = amphetamines and amphetamine-like substances.
*Only use not under a doctor's orders included.

Source: National Institute on Drug Abuse, National High School Senior Survey: "Monitoring the Future," 1989

NATIONAL HIGH SCHOOL SENIOR SURVEY, 1975-1989

High School Senior Survey
Trends in Lifetime Prevalence
Percent Who Ever Used

Class of 1980	Class of 1981	Class of 1982	Class of 1983	Class of 1984	Class of 1985	Class of 1986	Class of 1987	Class of 1988	Class of 1989
60.3	59.5	58.7	57.0	54.9	54.2	50.9	50.2	47.2	43.7
11.9	12.3	12.8	13.6	14.4	15.4	15.9	17.0	16.7	17.6
17.3	17.2	17.7	18.2	18.0	18.1	20.1	18.6	17.5	18.6
11.1	10.1	9.8	8.4	8.1	7.9	8.6	4.7	3.2	3.3
13.3	13.3	12.5	11.9	10.7	10.3	9.7	10.3	8.9	9.4
15.6	15.3	14.3	13.6	12.3	12.1	11.9	10.6	9.2	9.9
9.3	9.8	9.6	8.9	8.0	7.5	7.2	8.4	7.7	8.3
9.6	7.8	6.0	5.6	5.0	4.9	4.8	3.0	2.9	3.9
15.7	16.5	16.0	16.2	16.1	17.3	16.9	15.2	12.1	10.3
NA	NA	NA	NA	NA	NA	NA	5.4	4.8	4.7
NA	NA	NA	NA	NA	NA	NA	14.0	12.1	8.5
1.1	1.1	1.2	1.2	1.3	1.2	1.1	1.2	1.1	1.3
9.8	10.1	9.6	9.4	9.7	10.2	9.0	9.2	8.6	8.3
26.4	32.2	35.6	35.4	NA	NA	NA	NA	NA	NA
NA	NA	27.9	26.9	27.9	26.2	23.4	21.6	19.8	19.1
14.9	16.0	15.2	14.4	13.3	11.8	10.4	8.7	7.8	7.4
11.0	11.3	10.3	9.9	9.9	9.2	8.4	7.4	6.7	6.5
9.5	10.6	10.7	10.1	8.3	6.7	5.2	4.0	3.3	2.7
15.2	14.7	14.0	13.3	12.4	11.9	10.9	10.9	9.4	7.6
93.2	92.6	92.8	92.6	92.6	92.2	91.3	92.2	92.0	90.7
71.0	71.0	70.1	70.6	69.7	68.8	67.6	67.2	66.4	65.7

Appendix V

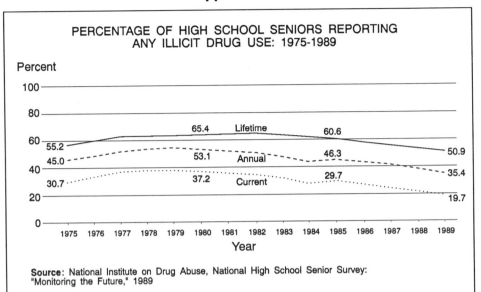

PERCENTAGE OF HIGH SCHOOL SENIORS REPORTING
ANY ILLICIT DRUG USE: 1975-1989

Percent

Source: National Institute on Drug Abuse, National High School Senior Survey:
"Monitoring the Future," 1989

Appendix VI

DRUG ABUSE AND AIDS

An estimated 25 percent of all cases of acquired immunodeficiency syndrome, or AIDS, are intravenous (IV) drug abusers. This group is the second largest at risk for AIDS, exceeded only by homosexual, and bisexual men. And the numbers may be growing. Data for the first half of 1988 show that IV drug abusers made up about 31 percent of the total reported cases.

". . . the number of IV drug users with AIDS is doubling every 14-16 months."

According to the National Institute on Drug Abuse (NIDA). There are 1.1 to 1.3 million IV drug users in the United States, and, so far, about 17,500 have developed AIDS. Thousands more are infected with the virus that causes this fatal illness, which kills by destroying the body's ability to fight disease.

Currently, the number of IV drug users with AIDS is doubling every 14-16 months. Although the numbers of IV drug users who carry the AIDS virus varies from region to region, in some places the majority may already be infected. In New York City, for example, 60 percent of IV drug users entering treatment programs have the AIDS virus.

Among IV drug abusers, the AIDS virus is spread primarily by needle sharing. As long as IV drug abusers are drug dependent, they are likely to engage in needle sharing. Thus, the key to eliminating needle sharing—and the associated spread of AIDS—is drug abuse treatment to curb drug dependence. NIDA is working to find ways to get more IV users into treatment and to develop new methods to fight drug addiction.

Most non-drug users characteristically associate heroin with IV drug use. However, thousands of others inject cocaine or amphetamines. Recent evidence suggests that IV cocaine use is increasing and that the AIDS virus is spreading in those users. One reason for this may be because cocaine's effects last only a short time. When the drug, which is a stimulant, wears off, users may inject again and again, sharing a needle many times in a few hours. In contrast, heroin users inject once and fall asleep.

". . . IV cocaine use is increasing and the AIDS virus is spreading in those users."

The apparent increase in IV cocaine is especially worrisome, drug abuse experts say, because there are no standard therapies for treating cocaine addiction. Until scientists find effective treatments for this problem, the ability to control the spread of AIDS will be hampered.

TRANSMISSION

Needle Sharing -- Among IV drug users, transmission of AIDS virus most often occurs by sharing needles, syringes, or other "works." Small amounts of contaminated blood left in the equipment can carry the virus from user to user. IV drug abusers who frequent "shooting galleries" — where paraphernalia is passed among several people -- are at especially high risk for AIDS. But, needle sharing of any sort (at parties, for example) can transmit the virus, and NIDA experts note that almost all IV drug users share needles at one time or another.

Because not every IV drug abuser will enter treatment and because some must wait to be treated, IV users in many cities are being taught to flush their "works" with bleach before they inject. Used correctly, bleach can destroy virus left in the equipment.

Sexual Transmission -- IV drug abusers also get AIDS through unprotected sex with someone who is infected. In addition, the AIDS virus can be sexually transmitted from infected IV drug abusers to individuals who do not use drugs. Data from the Centers for Disease Control show that IV drug use is associated with the increased spread of AIDS in the heterosexual population. For example, of all women reported to have AIDS, 49 percent were IV drug users, while another 30 percent -- non-IV drug users themselves -- were sexual partners of IV drug users. Infected women who become pregnant can pass the AIDS virus to their babies. About 70 percent of all children born with AIDS have had a mother or father who shot drugs.

Non-IV Drug Use and AIDS -- Sexual activity has also been reported as the means of AIDS transmission among those who use non-IV drugs (like crack or marijuana). Many people, especially women, addicted to crack (or other substances) go broke supporting their habit and turn to trading sex for drugs. Another link between substance abuse and AIDS is when individuals using alcohol and drugs relax their restraints and caution regarding sexual behavior. People who normally practice "safe" sex may neglect to do so while "under the influence."

Source: U.S. Public Health Service, AIDS Program Office, 1989

Appendix VII

U.S. Drug Schedules*

	Drugs Included	Dispensing Regulations
Schedule I high potential for abuse; no currently accepted medical use in treatment in U.S.; safety not proven for medical use	heroin methaqualone LSD mescaline peyote phencyclidine analogs psilocybin marijuana hashish	research use only
Schedule II high potential for abuse; currently accepted U.S. medical use; abuse may lead to severe psychological or physical dependence	opium morphine methadone barbiturates cocaine amphetamines phencyclidine codeine	written Rx; no refills
Schedule III less potential for abuse than drugs in Schedules I and II; currently accepted U.S. medical use; may lead to moderate or low physical dependence or high psychological dependence	glutethimide selected morphine, opium, and codeine compounds selected depressant sedative compounds selected stimulants for weight control	written or oral Rx; refills allowed
Schedule IV low potential for abuse relative to drugs in Schedule III; currently accepted U.S. medical use; abuse may lead to limited physical dependence or psychological dependence relative to drugs in Schedule III	selected barbiturate and other depressant compounds selected stimulants for weight control	written or oral Rx; refills allowed
Schedule V low potential for abuse relative to drugs in Schedule IV; currently accepted U.S. medical use; abuse may lead to limited physical dependence or psychological dependence relative to drugs in Schedule IV	selected narcotic compounds	OTC/ M.D.'s order

*Established by the U.S. Controlled Substances Act of 1970
Source: U.S. Drug Enforcement Administration

Appendix VIII

Agencies for the Prevention and Treatment of Drug Abuse

UNITED STATES

Alabama
Department of Mental Health
Division of Substance Abuse
200 Interstate Park Drive
P.O. Box 3710
Montgomery, AL 36109
(205) 270-9650

Alaska
Department of Health and
  Social Services
Division of Alcoholism and
  Drug Abuse
P.O. Box H
Juneau, AK 99811-0607
(907) 586-6201

Arizona
Department of Health
  Services
Division of Behavioral Health
  Services
Bureau of Community
  Services
The Office of Substance
  Abuse
2632 East Thomas
Phoenix, AZ 85016
(602) 255-1030

Arkansas
Department of Human
  Services
Division of Alcohol and Drug
  Abuse
400 Donagy Plaza North
P.O. Box 1437
Slot 2400
Little Rock, AR 72203-1437
(501) 682-6656

California
Health and Welfare Agencies
Department of Alcohol and
  Drug Programs
1700 K Street
Sacramento, CA 95814-4037
(916) 445-1943

Colorado
Department of Health
Alcohol and Drug Abuse
  Division
4210 East 11th Avenue
Denver, CO 80220
(303) 331-8201

Connecticut
Alcohol and Drug Abuse
  Commission
999 Asylum Avenue
3rd Floor
Hartford, CT 06105
(203) 566-4145

Delaware
Division of Mental Health
Bureau of Alcoholism and
  Drug Abuse
1901 North Dupont Highway
Newcastle, DE 19720
(302) 421-6101

District of Columbia
Department of Human
  Services
Office of Health Planning and
  Development
1660 L Street NW
Room 715
Washington, DC 20036
(202) 724-5641

Florida
Department of Health and
  Rehabilitative Services
Alcohol, Drug Abuse, and
  Mental Health Office
1317 Winewood Boulevard
Building 6, Room 183
Tallahassee, FL 32399-0700
(904) 488-8304

Georgia
Department of Human
  Resources
Division of Mental Health,
  Mental Retardation, and
  Substance Abuse
Alcohol and Drug Section
878 Peachtree Street
Suite 319
Atlanta, GA 30309-3917
(404) 894-4785

Hawaii
Department of Health
Mental Health Division
Alcohol and Drug Abuse
  Branch
1270 Queen Emma Street
Room 706
Honolulu, HI 96813
(808) 548-4280

Idaho
Department of Health and
  Welfare
Bureau of Preventive
  Medicine
Substance Abuse Section
450 West State
Boise, ID 83720
(208) 334-5934

Illinois
Department of Alcoholism
  and Substance Abuse
Illinois Center
100 West Randolph Street
Suite 5-600
Chicago, IL 60601
(312) 814-3840

Indiana
Department of Mental Health
Division of Addiction Services
117 East Washington Street
Indianapolis, IN 46204-3647
(317) 232-7816

Iowa
Department of Public Health
Division of Substance Abuse
Lucas State Office Building
321 East 12th Street
Des Moines, IA 50319
(515) 281-3641

Kansas
Department of Social
  Rehabilitation
Alcohol and Drug Abuse
  Services
300 SW Oakley
2nd Floor
Biddle Building
Topeka, KS 66606
(913) 296-3925

Kentucky
Cabinet for Human Resources
Department of Health
  Services
Substance Abuse Branch
275 East Main Street
Frankfort, KY 40621
(502) 564-2880

Louisiana
Department of Health and
  Hospitals
Office of Human Services
Division of Alcohol and Drug
  Abuse
P.O. Box 3868
Baton Rouge, LA 70821-3868
1201 Capital Access Road
Baton Rouge, LA 70802
(504) 342-9354

Maine
Department of Human
  Services
Office of Alcoholism and
  Drug Abuse Prevention
Bureau of Rehabilitation
5 Anthony Avenue
State House, Station 11
Augusta, ME 04433
(207) 289-2781

Maryland
Alcohol and Drug Abuse
  Administration
201 West Preston Street

4th Floor
Baltimore, MD 21201
(301) 225-6910

Massachusetts
Department of Public Health
Division of Substance Abuse
150 Tremont Street
Boston, MA 02111
(617) 727-1960

Michigan
Department of Public Health
Office of Substance Abuse
  Services
2150 Apollo Drive
P.O. Box 30206
Lansing, MI 48909
(517) 335-8810

Minnesota
Department of Human
  Services
Chemical Dependency
  Division
444 Lafayette Road
St. Paul, MN 55155
(612) 296-4614

Mississippi
Department of Mental Health
Division of Alcohol and Drug
  Abuse
1101 Robert E. Lee Building
239 North Lamar Street
Jackson, MS 39201
(601) 359-1288

Missouri
Department of Mental
  Health
Division of Alcoholism and
  Drug Abuse
1706 East Elm Street
P.O. Box 687
Jefferson City, MO 65102
(314) 751-4942

Montana
Department of Institutions
Alcohol and Drug Abuse
  Division
1539 11th Avenue
Helena, MT 59620
(406) 444-2827

Nebraska
Department of Public
  Institutions
Division of Alcoholism and
  Drug Abuse
801 West Van Dorn Street
P.O. Box 94728
Lincoln, NB 68509-4728
(402) 471-2851, Ext. 5583

Nevada
Department of Human
  Resources
Bureau of Alcohol and Drug
  Abuse
505 East King Street
Room 500
Carson City, NV 89710
(702) 687-4790

New Hampshire
Department of Health and
  Human Services
Office of Alcohol and Drug
  Abuse Prevention
State Office
Park South
105 Pleasant Street
Concord, NH 03301
(603) 271-6100

New Jersey
Department of Health
Division of Alcoholism and
  Drug Abuse
129 East Hanover Street CN
  362
Trenton, NJ 08625
(609) 292-8949

New Mexico
Health and Environment
  Department
Behavioral Health Services
  Division/
Substance Abuse
Harold Runnels Building
1190 Saint Francis Drive
Santa Fe, NM 87503
(505) 827-2601

New York
Division of Alcoholism and
  Alcohol Abuse
194 Washington Avenue

Albany, NY 12210
(518) 474-5417

Division of Substance Abuse
Services
Executive Park South
Box 8200
Albany, NY 12203
(518) 457-7629

North Carolina
Department of Human
Resources
Division of Mental Health,
Developmental Disabilities,
and Substance Abuse
Services
Alcohol and Drug Abuse
Services
325 North Salisbury Street
Albemarle Building
Raleigh, NC 27603
(919) 733-4670

North Dakota
Department of Human Services
Division of Alcohol and Drug
Abuse
1839 East Capital Avenue
Bismarck, ND 58501-2152
(701) 224-2769

Ohio
Division of Alcohol and Drug
Addiction Services
246 North High Street
3rd Floor
Columbus, OH 43266-0170
(614) 466-3445

Oklahoma
Department of Mental Health
and Substance Abuse
Services
Alcohol and Drug Abuse
Services
1200 North East 13th Street
P.O. Box 53277
Oklahoma City, OK 73152-
3277
(405) 271-8653

Oregon
Department of Human
Resources

Office of Alcohol and Drug
Abuse Programs
1178 Chemeketa NE
#102
Salem, OR 97310
(503) 378-2163

Pennsylvania
Department of Health
Office of Drug and Alcohol
Programs
Health and Welfare Building
Room 809
P.O. Box 90
Harrisburg, PA 17108
(717) 787-9857

Rhode Island
Department of Mental Health,
Mental Retardation and
Hospitals
Division of Substance Abuse
Substance Abuse
Administration Building
P.O. Box 20363
Cranston, RI 02920
(401) 464-2091

South Carolina
Commission on Alcohol and
Drug Abuse
3700 Forest Drive Suite 300
Columbia, SC 29204
(803) 734-9520

South Dakota
Department of Human
Services
700 Governor's Drive
Pier South D
Pierre, SD 57501-2291
(605) 773-4806

Tennessee
Department of Mental Health
and Mental Retardation
Alcohol and Drug Abuse
Services
706 Church Street
Nashville, TN 37243-0675
(615) 741-1921

Texas
Commission on Alcohol and
Drug Abuse

720 Bracos Street
Suite 403
Austin, TX 78701
(512) 463-5510

Utah
Department of Social Services
Division of Substance Abuse
120 North 200 West
4th Floor
Salt Lake City, UT 84103
(801) 538-3939

Vermont
Agency of Human Services
Department of Social and
Rehabilitation Services
Office of Alcohol and Drug
Abuse Programs
103 South Main Street
Waterbury, VT 05676
(802) 241-2170

Virginia
Department of Mental Health
and Mental Retardation
Division of Substance Abuse
109 Governor Street
8th Floor
P.O. Box 1797
Richmond, VA 23214
(804) 786-5313

Washington
Department of Social and
Health Service
Division of Alcohol and
Substance Abuse
12th and Franklin
Mail Stop OB 21W
Olympia, WA 98504
(206) 753-5866

West Virginia
Department of Health and
Human Resources
Office of Behavioral Health
Services
Division on Alcoholism and
Drug Abuse
Capital Complex
1900 Kanawha Boulevard East
Building 3, Room 402
Charleston, WV 25305
(304) 348-2276

Wisconsin

Department of Health and
Social Services
Division of Community
Services
Bureau of Community
Programs
Office of Alcohol and Drug
Abuse
1 West Wilson Street
P.O. Box 7851
Madison, WI 53707-7851
(608) 266-2717

Wyoming

Alcohol And Drug Abuse
Programs
451 Hathaway Building
Cheyenne, WY 82002
(307) 777-7115

U.S. TERRITORIES AND POSSESSIONS

American Samoa

LBJ Tropical Medical Center
Department of Mental Health
Clinic
Pago Pago, American Samoa
96799

Guam

Mental Health & Substance
Abuse Agency
P.O. Box 20999
Guam 96921

Puerto Rico

Department of Addiction
Control Services
Alcohol and Drug Abuse
Programs
Avenida Barbosa
P.O. Box 414
Rio Piedras, PR 00928-1474
(809) 763-7575

Trust Territories

Director of Health Services
Office of the High
Commissioner
Saipan, Trust Territories
96950

Virgin Islands

Division of Health and
Substance Abuse
Becastro Building
3rd Street, Sugar Estate
St. Thomas, Virgin Islands
00802

CANADA

Canadian Centre on
Substance Abuse
112 Kent Street, Suite 480
Ottawa, Ontario
K1P 5P2
(613) 235-4048

Alberta

Alberta Alcohol and Drug
Abuse Commission
10909 Jasper Avenue, 6th
Floor
Edmonton, Alberta
T5J 3M9
(403) 427-2837

British Columbia

Ministry of Labour and
Consumer Services
Alcohol and Drug Programs
1019 Wharf Street, 5th Floor
Victoria, British Columbia
V8V 1X4
(604) 387-5870

Manitoba

The Alcoholism Foundation of
Manitoba
1031 Portage Avenue
Winnipeg, Manitoba
R3G 0R8
(204) 944-6226

New Brunswick

Alcoholism and Drug
Dependency Commission
of New Brunswick
65 Brunswick Street
P.O. Box 6000
Fredericton, New Brunswick
E3B 5H1
(506) 453-2136

Newfoundland

The Alcohol and Drug
Dependency Commission
of Newfoundland and
Labrador
Suite 105, Prince Charles
Building
120 Torbay Road, 1st Floor
St. John's, Newfoundland
A1A 2G8
(709) 737-3600

Northwest Territories

Alcohol and Drug Services
Department of Social
Services
Government of Northwest
Territories
Box 1320 - 52nd Street
6th Floor, Precambrian
Building
Yellowknife, Northwest
Territories
S1A 2L9
(403) 920-8005

Nova Scotia

Nova Scotia Commission on
Drug Dependency
6th Floor, Lord Nelson
Building
5675 Spring Garden Road
Halifax, Nova Scotia
B3J 1H1
(902) 424-4270

Ontario

Addiction Research
Foundation
33 Russell Street
Toronto, Ontario
M5S 2S1
(416) 595-6000

Prince Edward Island

Addiction Services of Prince
Edward Island
P.O. Box 37
Eric Found Building
65 McGill Avenue
Charlottetown, Prince Edward
Island
C1A 7K2
(902) 368-4120

Quebec

Service des Programmes aux
    Personnes Toxicomanie
Gouvernement du Quebec
Ministere de la Sante et des
    Services Sociaux
1005 Chemin Ste. Foy
Quebec City, Quebec
G1S 4N4
(418) 643-9887

Saskatchewan

Saskatchewan Alcohol and
    Drug Abuse Commission
1942 Hamilton Street
Regina, Saskatchewan
S4P 3V7
(306) 787-4085

Yukon

Alcohol and Drug Services
Department of Health and
    Social Resources
Yukon Territorial
    Government
6118-6th Avenue
P.O. Box 2703
Whitehorse, Yukon Territory
Y1A 2C6
(403) 667-5777

Further Reading

General

Berger, Gilda. *Drug Abuse: The Impact on Society.* New York: Watts, 1988. (Gr. 7–12)

Cohen, Susan, and Daniel Cohen. *What You Can Believe About Drugs: An Honest and Unhysterical Guide for Teens.* New York: M. Evans, 1987. (Gr. 7–12)

Musto, David F. *The American Disease: Origins of Narcotic Control.* Rev. ed. New Haven: Yale University Press, 1987.

National Institute on Drug Abuse. *Drug Use, Drinking, and Smoking: National Survey Results from High School, College, and Young Adult Populations, 1975–1988.* Washington, DC: Public Health Service, Department of Health and Human Services, 1989.

O'Brien, Robert, and Sidney Cohen. *Encyclopedia of Drug Abuse.* New York: Facts on File, 1984.

Snyder, Solomon H., M.D. *Drugs and the Brain.* New York: Scientific American Books, 1986.

U.S. Department of Justice. *Drugs of Abuse.* 1989 edition. Washington, DC: Government Printing Office, 1989.

PCP

Journal of Psychedelic Drugs (January–June 1978). Entire issue devoted to PCP.

McNichol, Tom. "PCP: The Cheap Thrill with a High Price." *Rolling Stone* (March 24, 1988).

Miller, N. S., et al. "PCP: A Dangerous Drug." *American Family Physician* (September 1988).

Stafford, Peter. *Psychedelics Encyclopedia.* Rev. ed. Los Angeles: Tarcher, 1983.

Thombs, D. L. "A Review of PCP Abuse Trends and Perceptions." *Public Health Report* (July–August 1989).

Glossary

AIDS   acquired immune deficiency syndrome; an acquired defect in the immune system; the final stage of the disease caused by the human immunodeficiency virus (HIV); spread by the exchange of blood (including contaminated hypodermic needles), by sexual contact, through nutritive fluids passed from a mother to her fetus, and through breast-feeding; leaves victims vulnerable to certain, often fatal, infections and cancers

amnesia   a permanent or temporary loss of memory

amphetamines   drugs that stimulate the nervous system, generally used as mood elevators, energizers, antidepressants, appetite depressants, and as substances to increase alertness and activity

analgesia   insensitivity to pain without loss of consciousness

analog   a drug that is similar to another drug in both chemical structure and function

anesthetic   a drug that produces loss of sensation, sometimes with loss of consciousness

antagonist   a drug that blocks or counteracts the effects of another drug

antidepressant   a drug that elevates the mood

antidote   same as antagonist

antipsychotic   a drug that calms a person who is in a psychotic state

ataxia   loss of coordination

bad trip   an unwanted experience caused by a drug

barbiturates   drugs that cause depression of the central nervous system, generally used to reduce anxiety or to induce euphoria

behavioral tolerance   the process whereby a drug user learns to compensate for, or to overcome, a drug's disruptive effects on normal behavior

catatonic   a state characterized by muscle rigidity and stupor, sometimes alternating with excitement and confusion

cocaine   a stimulant made from the leaves of the coca plant

coma   a state of prolonged unconsciousness

convulsions   contortions of the body caused by violent muscular contractions of the extremities, trunk, and head

delusional   not grounded in reality

dissociative anesthetic   a drug, such as PCP and ketamine, that produces distortions of body image and feelings of separation from the environment *drug* any substance, plant, powder, solid, fluid, or gas that when ingested, injected, sniffed, inhaled, or absorbed from the skin affects bodily functions

drug interaction a change in the action of one drug by earlier or simultaneous administration of another drug

euphoria a feeling of well-being or elation

hallucination a sensory impression that has no basis in reality

hallucinogen an agent capable of producing hallucinations

Haldo an antipsychotic used during PCP treatment

heroin a semisynthetic opiate produced by a chemical modification of morphine

intoxication an effect of a drug characterized by marked changes or impairment in behavior

ketamine a surgical anesthetic that is similar to, but much less potent than, PCP

LSD lysergic acid diethylamide; an organic compound that induces psychotic symptoms similar to those of schizophrenia

marijuana a hemp plant that contains THC, a habit-forming intoxicating drug

mescaline a hallucinogenic drug chemically similar to amphetamine, found in certain cacti

methohexital a type of sedative

morphine the major sedative and pain-relieving drug found in opium

narcotic originally, a group of drugs producing effects similar to morphine; often used to refer to any substance that sedates, has a depressive effect, and/or causes dependence

neurological pertaining to the nervous system

neuron one of the cells that comprise the nervous system

opiate any drug whose effects on the body are similar to those caused by morphine

overdose when more of a drug is taken than the amount necessary to obtain a desired effect, usually resulting in adverse effects or even death

paranoid suffering from extreme suspiciousness and/or fear

paraphernalia the equipment and material used to administer or store illicit drugs

pathological due to or involving a mental or physical disease

pentobarbital a short-acting barbiturate

pharmacology the study of drugs, their sources, preparations, and uses

physical dependence an adaptation of the body to the presence of a drug to the extent that withdrawal from the drug produces unpleasant physiological symptoms

physiological tolerance   tolerance caused by heightened sensitivity to a drug at brain receptor sites or by increased rate of metabolism and excretion of a drug due to an increased production of enzymes

potency   a measure of a drug's activity in terms of how much of it is needed to produce a given effect; the lower the dose required to produce the desired effect, the more potent the drug

psilocybin   an LSD-like drug that alters sensory perception

psychedelic drug   a drug with the ability to alter sensory perception

psychoactive drug   a drug that alters mood and/or behavior

psychological dependence   a condition in which the drug user craves a drug to maintain a sense of well-being and feels emotional discomfort when deprived of the drug

psychosis   a major emotional disorder characterized by derangement of the personality and loss of contact with reality, often with delusions, hallucinations, or illusions

run   a prolonged period of drug use

schizophrenia   a chronic psychotic disorder whose predominant symptoms are paranoia, delusions, and hallucinations

sedative-hypnotic drug   a drug that produces a general depressant effect on the nervous system

stereotyped behavior   behavior characterized by repetitive movements

subjective effects   the action of a drug on a person's moods, thoughts, feelings, sensations, and/or perceptions

THC   tetra-hydrocannabinol, the psychoactive ingredient in marijuana

therapeutic ratio   the fatal dosage of a drug divided by the smallest dosage necessary to produce the desired effect; a measure of drug safety

tolerance   a decrease of susceptibility to the effects of a drug due to its continued administration, resulting in the user's need to increase the drug dosage in order to achieve the effects experienced previously

toxic effect   a drug-induced condition that is temporarily or permanently damaging to cells or organ systems of the body

tranquilizer   a drug that has calming, relaxing effects

withdrawal   the physiological and psychological effects of discontinued usage of a drug

Index

Marilyn Carroll, Ph.D., received her degree in psychology from Florida State University and teaches in the Department of Psychiatry at the University of Minnesota. She was a research fellow at the University of Minnesota and held a National Research Service Award. She has also served as president of ISGIDAR, an international group of scientists studying basic properties of psychoactive drugs.

Paul R. Sanberg, Ph.D., is a professor of psychiatry, psychology, neurosurgery, physiology, and biophysics at the University of Cincinnati College of Medicine. Currently, he is also a professor of psychiatry at Brown University and scientific director for Cellular Transplants, Inc., in Providence, Rhode Island.

Professor Sanberg has held research positions at the Australian National University at Canberra, the Johns Hopkins University School of Medicine, and Ohio University. He has written many journal articles and book chapters in the fields of neuroscience and psychopharmacology. He has served on the editorial boards of many scientific journals and is the recipient of numerous awards.

Solomon H. Snyder, M.D., is Distinguished Service Professor of Neuroscience, Pharmacology and Psychiatry at the Johns Hopkins University School of Medicine. He has served as president of the Society for Neuroscience and in 1978 received the Albert Lasker Award in Medical Research. He has authored *Drugs and the Brain, Uses of Marijuana, Madness and the Brain, The Troubled Mind,* and *Biological Aspects of Mental Disorder* and has edited *Perspectives in Neuropharmacology: A Tribute to Julius Axelrod.* Professor Snyder was a research associate with Dr. Axelrod at the National Institutes of Health.

Barry L. Jacobs, Ph.D., is currently a professor in the neuroscience program at Princeton University. Professor Jacobs is the author of *Serotonin Neurotransmission and Behavior* and *Hallucinogens: Neurochemical, Behavioral and Clinical Perspectives.* He has written many journal articles in the field of neuroscience and contributed numerous chapters to books on behavior and brain science. He has been a member of several panels of the National Institute of Mental Health.

Jerome H. Jaffe, M.D., formerly professor of psychiatry at the College of Physicians and Surgeons, Columbia University, is director of the Addiction Research Center of the National Institute on Drug Abuse. Dr. Jaffe is also a psychopharmacologist and has conducted research on a wide range of addictive drugs and developed treatment programs for addicts. He has acted as special consultant to the president on narcotics and dangerous drugs and was the first director of the White House Special Action Office for Drug Abuse Prevention.